TABLE OF CONTENTS

Top 20 Test Taking Tips

1. Carefully follow all the test registration procedures
2. Know the test directions, duration, topics, question types, how many questions
3. Setup a flexible study schedule at least 3-4 weeks before test day
4. Study during the time of day you are most alert, relaxed, and stress free
5. Maximize your learning style; visual learner use visual study aids, auditory learner use auditory study aids
6. Focus on your weakest knowledge base
7. Find a study partner to review with and help clarify questions
8. Practice, practice, practice
9. Get a good night's sleep; don't try to cram the night before the test
10. Eat a well balanced meal
11. Know the exact physical location of the testing site; drive the route to the site prior to test day
12. Bring a set of ear plugs; the testing center could be noisy
13. Wear comfortable, loose fitting, layered clothing to the testing center; prepare for it to be either cold or hot during the test
14. Bring at least 2 current forms of ID to the testing center
15. Arrive to the test early; be prepared to wait and be patient
16. Eliminate the obviously wrong answer choices, then guess the first remaining choice
17. Pace yourself; don't rush, but keep working and move on if you get stuck
18. Maintain a positive attitude even if the test is going poorly
19. Keep your first answer unless you are positive it is wrong
20. Check your work, don't make a careless mistake

Trauma

Brain Injury

Patients sustaining traumatic brain injury and a Glasgow coma scale ranking between 13 and 15 are said to have mild injury. However, many of these patients may not even be seen by a doctor. Transient unsteadiness and confusion may accompany mild traumatic brain injury. Most will feel well within minutes, but signs of secondary injury should be monitored. Written descriptions of these signs and instructions of what to do if they develop should be provided for the patient and their support person. Categories of mildly injured patients that should be observed include those with drainage of cerebral spinal fluid from the ear or nose, and those who have consumed alcohol, drugs, or have a medical condition that interferes with neurological assessment.

Patients sustaining traumatic brain injury and a Glasgow coma scale ranking between 9 and 12 are said to have moderate injury. In these cases, the nervous system trauma is often deemed of secondary urgency relative to other concurrent problems. However, initial treatment should reflect that provided to severely injured patients, including assumption of cervical spinal injury until ruled otherwise. Neurological monitoring is of continued importance to quickly address signs of deterioration. These patients are at risk for anxiety and depression, as well as the long term problems that make up post-concussion syndrome, such as fatigue, irritability, headache, and forgetfulness. Providing information and support to help patients prepare for and cope with these issues can help them minimize the negative impact of the injury on home or work life.

Traumatic brain injury may compromise blood vessel integrity, leading to hemorrhage and hematoma. If the hemorrhage occurs in the subdural space between the dura mater and arachnoid layers, it causes a subdural hematoma. Hemorrhage may be evident immediately following trauma, but slow developing chronic hematomas may not manifest clinically until months later. Early detection prevents possible compression, mass effect, and ischemia. Acute subdural hematomas are composed of clotted blood, whereas chronic subdural hematomas are made up of fluid blood. Symptoms of chronic subdural hematoma may develop slowly, and include headache, confusion, and drowsiness. The elderly are particularly susceptible due to strain on bridging veins between neural tissue and the dura, and natural brain shrinkage that leaves more space for blood to accumulate before symptoms develop.

Primary traumatic brain injury is insult caused directly by contact to the head and brain at the time of injury. Contact phenomena injuries are caused by impact with the head. Low velocity impact limits injury to the scalp (laceration) or skull (fracture), whereas high velocity impact involves the brain as well (intracerebral hemorrhage). A difference between inertia of the brain and skull causes compression and tension during an abrupt stoppage of motion. Such acceleration-deceleration injury may occur in the antero-postero direction, damaging the frontal or temporal lobes, or rotational acceleration-deceleration may cause shearing between cerebral and connective tissue. The inferior surfaces of the frontal and temporal lobes are also susceptible to injurious contact with the bones at the base of the skull.

Primary brain injury induces damaging secondary brain injury events including intracranial hemorrhage, cerebral edema, and increased intracranial pressure. Multisystem complications also arise, including hypotension, respiratory problems, infection, and electrolyte imbalance. These conditions in turn precipitate further injury. Cerebral swelling may be general or localized and caused by edema (increased cerebral water content), or by increased cerebral blood volume. Brain swelling or intracranial hematoma can increase intracranial pressure, increasing likelihood of mass effect and herniation. Blunt trauma patients with high intracranial pressure or low blood pressure are more likely to sustain hypoxia and ischemia, which can lead to coma. Secondary injuries are generally considered to develop four hours or more later than the initial injury, and a major goal of primary care is to minimize their occurrence.

Until ruled otherwise, patients with moderate to severe traumatic brain injury should be treated as though the injury is severe. Likewise, conservative neck and spine care should be exercised until possible damage is assessed. Patients sustaining traumatic brain injury and a Glasgow coma scale ranking between 3 and 8 are said to have severe injury. Stabilization and resuscitation treatments in the emergency department are of primary importance. Following emergency department care, severely injured patients may undergo surgery or be admitted directly to the ICU, where monitoring of intracranial pressure and cerebral oxygenation is continued. Low level of consciousness is linked with more extensive damage, increased risk of secondary injury, and poor outcome.

Traumatic brain injury produces a range of complications in various bodily systems. Assuring respiratory or ventilator function and airway patency are critical. Positioning the patient on their side facilitates drainage, and suctioning clears the airway. Atelectasis, or reduced functional lung volume, can be prevented with chest physical therapy or deep breathing exercises. These measures also prevent aspiration and pneumonia. Cardiovascular function should be monitored for cardiac arrhythmias and to maintain appropriate blood pressure. Immobility leads to deep vein thrombosis and pulmonary emboli. Elastic stockings, compression boots and heparin may be used to prevent clot formation. Antacids or other drugs may be used to control gastric pH, thereby preventing irritation, ulcers, and gastrointestinal hemorrhage. Use of higher saline concentrations for fluid replacement can help prevent hyponatremia (low blood sodium concentration), which can lead to seizure or coma. Hyperglycemia should be prevented with insulin, as it may worsen ischemic injury. Nutritional needs should be assessed by a dietitian and addressed as soon as possible with a feeding tube inserted in the jejunum.

Four types of blast injury

Traumatic brain injury caused by blast exposure is manifested by four types of blast injury. (1) Overpressurization or a complex pressure wave results in a primary blast injury, which may target air-filled organs of the ear, lung, and gastrointestinal tract, as well as fluid-filled cavities of the brain and spinal cord. (2) When energized fragments fly through the air, a secondary blast injury can occur. (3) A tertiary blast injury, or blunt force trauma, takes place during a motor vehicle accident at high speed with acceleration or deceleration or when individuals are thrown into a solid object, such as a steering wheel. (4) The fourth type of blast injury can be caused by a severe form of blast trauma, such as toxic gas inhalation with an explosion or traumatic amputation with increased blood loss. It is very important to consider the mechanism of injury during an examination when distinguishing the physical, emotional, cognitive, and behavioral symptoms.

Treatment of a blast injury

Early treatment of cognitive deficits produces the best long-term results after a blast injury, leading to a complete recovery in the first year after the injury. There are three types of treatment options, including pharmacotherapy, patient education, and cognitive rehabilitation. If provided within 1–2 weeks post–blunt injury, patient education and support decreased somatic and psychological complaints. It appears that when patients with traumatic brain injuries were given educational literature about common symptoms and positive coping strategies within 1 week of the injury, these patients had fewer sleep and anxiety complaints than controls given no interventions. Speech–language pathologists typically provide this education, which includes coping strategies and positive recovery expectations. Data are limited on the effectiveness of cognitive rehabilitation; however, treatment for attention, memory function, and cognitive processing speed, resulted in neuropsychological improvement. Finally, treatment for attention deficits has been shown to be effective for direct attention training.

Proper emergency medical services triage for a blast injury

Proper emergency medical services triage for a blast injury involves multiple factors before transport, including the following: (1) the type and size of explosion; (2) the time of the explosion; (3) the proximity of the patient to the center of the blast; (4) any displacement of the patient by the blast wind; (5) any entrapment reports in collapsed structures; and (6) any presence of smoke, dust, secondary fire, or contamination by chemical or radioactive substances. The reduction of heat loss and prevention of hypothermia are essential. External hemorrhage should be identified to control life-threatening bleeding, such as with tourniquets, before transport. Should respiratory distress, thoracic trauma, or any abnormal auscultation findings be present, high-flow oxygen must be administered. If radioactive material is found by the use of a hand-held Geiger counter, the receiving hospital must be notified, and all personnel and equipment must be decontaminated.

Blunt traumatic brain injury

Blunt traumatic brain injury (TBI) is typically the result of motor vehicle accidents, involving cars, trucks, motorcycles, bicycles, and pedestrians; falls; violent acts, such as assaults; and injuries that occur during sporting activities. There are five related mechanisms of injury that have an impact on the outcome of blunt TBI. (1) Deceleration force involves an individual's head striking an immovable object. (2) Acceleration force involves a moving object striking an individual's head. (3) Due to rapid velocity changes within the cranial vault, injuries may occur from a combination of acceleration/deceleration forces. (4) Rotational forces are the result of a side-to-side and twisting movement within the cranial vault. Brain tissue tension and shearing are the result of the rotational injuries due to acceleration/deceleration forces. (5) Direct blows to the head that deform the skull result in brain tissue compression, which is also related to the impact velocity.

Treatment for blunt traumatic brain injury

In 2008, a study was conducted to determine the benefit and safety of administering enoxaparin for venous thromboembolism in patients with blunt traumatic brain injury (TBI); it concluded that enoxaparin was considered a viable treatment option for patients with blunt TBI when administered within 48 hours of admission and for TBI patients with additional risks for traumatic injury. In addition to the reduction of deep venous thrombosis and pulmonary embolism, there is likely to be a low risk of developing intracranial bleeding complications, such as progression of hemorrhage, apart from neurologic deterioration. Measurable outcomes included intracranial

- 7 -

bleeding complications, Glasgow Outcome Score at discharge, and hospital mortality. The enoxaparin protocol appeared to allow for early, safe, and effective prophylaxis in TBI patients.

Treatment for blunt traumatic brain injury in pediatric patients
Following minor head trauma, patients younger than 2 years are shown to be at a high risk for skull fracture and intracranial injury. Because of barriers to assessing this age-group fully, clinicians follow conservative approaches to diagnostic imaging, such as computed tomography (CT) imaging, as the potential risks from radiation exposure promote the selective use of CT scans. Therefore, CT scans are prudently recommended for pediatric patients felt to be at high risk for blunt traumatic brain injury. When diagnosed with postconcussion syndrome, bed rest alone does not result in an improved outcome. Education and multidisciplinary intervention, such as physical therapy or behavioral therapy, and concussion-specific follow-up therapy, such as those designed for tension-type headaches or migraines, may alleviate associated disabilities. Recommended pharmacologic management of postconcussive headaches involves nonsteroidal anti-inflammatory medication. In addition, research is underway to study the effectiveness of occipital nerve blocks, corticosteroids, and hyperbaric oxygen therapy.

Penetrating traumatic brain injury

Penetrating traumatic brain injury (TBI) is the result of impalement injuries, such as gunshot wounds, stab wounds, and nail guns. Three main events take place following a cranial missile injury. (1) Destruction of the local parenchyma occurs along the bullet track, which plays a major role in the extent of the injury. If the bullet is unable to exit the skull, it may ricochet, creating second and third tracks. (2) After the bullet enters the skull, shock and heat waves immediately develop and transmit throughout the intracranial cavity. Shock waves can lead to temporary or permanent medullary failure and cardiopulmonary arrest. (3) Parallel to the bullet track, a temporary cavity is created, which immediately collapses. Hematoma formation or pseudoaneurysm development may result from laceration of major cerebral vessels. Stab wounds to the head are often accompanied by neurologic symptoms from cerebral vessel laceration and hematoma formation.

Treatment of penetrating traumatic brain injury
In 1995, guidelines for the treatment of penetrating traumatic brain injury (TBI) were established by the Brain Trauma Foundation, which outlined the best practices to increase survival post-TBI. Emergency medical protocol prescribes the use of less oxygen pressure, as oxygen may decrease blood flow to the brain. Previously, intravenous (IV) fluids were not administered to TBI patients because of concerns about brain swelling; however, IV-fluid administration is now recommended. Monitoring blood pressure is vital to assess for any changes before fatal consequences develop. The operative procedure, decompressive craniectomy, has become a safe, effective, and accepted procedure. This procedure increases the potential volume of the cranial cavity by removing a large area of skull. Furthermore, time spent removing all of the foreign debris and fragments seemed to result in more near-fatal and fatal complications. After decompressive craniectomy was adopted in 1995, deaths from penetrating TBI decreased from 55% to 20%.

Surgical treatment of penetrating traumatic brain injury
Significant factors indicating the necessity of surgical treatment of penetrating traumatic brain injury include: (1) the removal of epidural, subdural, or intracerebral hematomas; (2) the removal of necrotic brain tissue; (3) the prevention of further ischemia and swelling; (4) the control of any active hemorrhage; (5) and the removal of bone fragments, metal, or other foreign bodies to prevent infection. The age of the patient, the location of the hematoma, and the patient's clinical

condition must be considered. The temporal region and the posterior fossa typically indicate aggressive treatment, as hematomas and contusions in these areas are known to herniate more frequently. Depending on the velocity of the bullet fragments or missiles and the size of the penetration, it is thought that fragments should not be removed unless accessible. Fragments are not strongly associated with infection; however, some metals may cause electrolysis, leading to fibroglial scarring and secondary epilepsy, and some fragments may migrate.

Epidural hematoma

An epidural hematoma, or extradural hemorrhage, may be caused by a skull fracture following a severe head injury, for example, after a motor vehicle or motorcycle accident. This results in an arterial or venous blood vessel rupture or tear, which bleeds into the cavity between the skull and the dura mater. A hematoma is formed by rapid bleeding, increasing intracranial pressure, which can lead to permanent brain damage and, if untreated, death. Because the membrane surrounding the brain is less firmly attached to the skull in young patients, extradural hemorrhage is more common in this age-group as compared to old patients. Symptoms of an extradural hemorrhage, which may occur minutes to hours following injury, include confusion, dizziness, drowsiness, unilateral pupil enlargement, severe headache, nausea, vomiting, weakness of the opposite side of the body from the dilated pupil, and a pattern of loss of consciousness (LOC) to alertness to rapid LOC.

Treatment for epidural hematoma
Epidural hematoma is defined as blood accumulation in the space between the bone and dura, either intracranial or spinal. Medication regimens are important in managing epidural hematomas. Osmotic diuretics, such as mannitol or hypertonic saline, diminish intracranial pressure by reversing the pressure gradient across the blood–brain barrier. Antipyretics, such as acetaminophen, are used to reduce the fever of hyperthermia, eliminating exacerbation of the neurological injury. To reduce the frequency of early post-traumatic seizures from cortical damage, anticonvulsants are used. If spinal cord decompression is involved with the spinal epidural hematoma, high-dose methylprednisolone is given, as tissue damage is mitigated by anti-inflammatory properties. Heparin is administered for the prevention of venous thrombosis in immobilized patients. To restore the patient's normal coagulation parameters, thereby reversing coagulopathies or bleeding diatheses, protamine and vitamin K are given. Antacids aid in preventing gastric ulcers that are associated with spinal cord damage and traumatic brain injury.

Surgical treatment of an epidural hematoma
Surgical treatment of an epidural hematoma involves the definitive surgical evacuation of the hematoma, as compared to conservative management. Preoperatively, a computed tomography (CT) scan demonstrates the location. The surgical procedure involves the following steps: (1) a craniotomy or laminectomy, (2) evacuation of the hematoma, (3) coagulation of the bleeding sites, (4) inspection of the dura, (5) tenting of the dura to the bone, and (6) insertion of epidural drains for up to 24 hours. Postoperatively, a CT scan is obtained to ensure that optimal evacuation of the intracranial hematoma has occurred. For nonsurgical candidates, minimally invasive procedures, still surgical, may be considered, including the use of burr holes and negative pressure drainage. Research is underway to determine the effectiveness of additional interventions, such as thrombolytic evacuation with a closed suction drain and endovascular embolization. The latter technique ensures minimal bleeding in the acute stage of the epidural hematoma.

Diffuse axonal injury

Diffuse axonal injury (DAI), otherwise known as axonal shearing or tearing, is a primary injury, resulting from traumatic deceleration in high-speed motor vehicle accidents and violent events. Axons are the long, communicating fibers for the neurons within the brain and central nervous system. A DAI can lead to a persistent vegetative state. Secondary factors, or the delayed component of the injury, also occur, including secondary swelling and retraction bulb formation. Mild DAIs involve loss of consciousness for 6–24 hours. Moderate DAIs typically are the result of basal skull fractures and can involve a comatose state for up to 24 hours. Severe DAIs typically involve primary brain stem injuries. Symptoms of DAI vary based on the location and severity of the tearing and also may be temporary or permanent. Symptoms may include cognitive impairment, fever, high blood pressure, muscle rigidity, coma, and death.

Treatment for diffuse axonal injury

Diffuse axonal injury (DAI) is a very debilitating closed head injury, which can lead to vegetative states or comas in 90% of patients. Treatment for severe closed head injury includes surgery to drain clotted blood and to accommodate brain swelling. Intracranial pressure is also relieved by diuretics, coma-inducing drugs, and antiseizure medication, thereby preventing further brain damage. Rehabilitation following surgery and medication management include therapy to regain cognitive and basic motor skills, continuing into the outpatient setting. Cognitive rehabilitation assists in restoring lost brain function, teaching the patient to compensate for brain functions that will not typically be restored. In addition, basic skills, such as focus, attention, and perception, are strengthened, followed by the addition of complex skills, such as reasoning, planning, and judgment. Neuropsychologists and physical therapists play an active role in the overall team that cares for patients, helping them to regain or manage lost skills.

Physical rehabilitation for diffuse axonal injury

When a patient suffering from a diffuse axonal injury demonstrates improvement after cognitive rehabilitation, such as attention, focus, and memory, assisted by cognitive and speech therapists, physical rehabilitation may be initiated. The purpose of physical rehabilitation is to restore the patient's physical function and to compensate for any physical impairment. Initially, simple movements, such as sitting, standing, and distinguishing between left and right, are taught and relearned. Subsequently, a patient is taught fine motor skills to perform the activities of daily living, such as eating, bathing, and tooth brushing. Physical rehabilitation is best done at a specialized traumatic brain injury treatment center, which has state-of-the-art equipment and is staffed by a specialized team, including physicians who are trained in neurology and physiatry, neuropsychologists, physical therapists, occupational therapists, and social workers.

Four types of skull fractures

There are four types of skull fractures: (1) A simple fracture involves a break with no skin damage. (2) A thin-line fracture, or linear skull fracture, does not involve bone distortion, depression, or splintering. (3) A depressed skull fracture involves a crushed area of the skull bone, pressing toward the brain. (4) Bone splintering with a break in the skin describes a compound fracture. Skull fractures are most commonly caused by head trauma from falls, physical assault, sport injuries, and automobile accidents. Symptoms can vary widely from a bump on the head with bruising within 24 hours, to severe symptoms, including bleeding from the wound, ears, nose, or periorbital area; bruises under the eyes or behind the ears; pupil changes; confusion; convulsions; balance difficulties; clear or bloody drainage from the nose or ears; drowsiness; headache; loss of consciousness; nausea or vomiting; irritability or restlessness; slurred speech; stiff neck; swelling; and vision changes.

Treatment for skull fractures

If neurologically intact, adults with simple linear skull fractures may be discharged and instructed to return to the hospital if symptoms occur; infants with simple linear fractures may be observed overnight. Linear basilar fractures are treated conservatively without antibiotics. Similarly, temporal bone fractures are treated conservatively, as the tympanic membrane will likely heal on its own. Simple depressed fractures in neurologically stable infants typically smooth out over time; seizure medications should be prescribed if the seizure risk rises above 20%. With open skull fractures, antibiotics, such as sulfisoxazole, and tetanus toxoid may be required if the fracture is contaminated. Conservative treatment for types I and II occipital condylar fractures includes neck stabilization with a hard collar, such as the Philadelphia collar, or halo traction. As surgical intervention is limited, immediate elevation of depressed skull fractures is indicated with gross contamination, dural tear with pneumocephalus, and an underlying hematoma. Additionally, craniectomy, followed by cranioplasty, and atlantoaxial arthrodesis may be indicated.

Ossiculoplasty for the treatment of a skull base fracture

Surgical intervention to treat ossicular incongruences as a result a longitudinal skull base fracture of the temporal bone is limited. Indications for ossiculoplasty, the reconstruction of the ossicular chain (i.e., recreation of the middle ear mechanism for sound conduction), include the following: (1) persistent hearing loss longer than 3 months, (2) nonhealing of the tympanic membrane, or (3) the presence of a persistent cerebrospinal fluid (CSF) leak. Preoperative detection of the CSF leak is mandatory. Materials used for ossicular reconstruction or substitution include biologic materials, such as autograft or homograft ossicles; cortical bone, teeth, and cartilage; and alloplastic materials, classified as biocompatible, bioinert, or bioactive. Determination of the material to be used is dependent on the status of the ossicular remnants. Optimally, reconstruction with as much of the remaining ossicular chain as possible results in better hearing postoperatively.

Lumbar strain

Low back pain may result from lumbosacral musculoligamentous sprains and strains. Repetitive stress injuries, as seen in athletes, may involve lumbar strains, which are considered the most common back injury. Strains involve a partial or complete tear of the muscle–tendon unit, typically resulting from a forceful muscular stretch that creates a muscular contraction. Posterior spinal muscles with associated tendons that cover several joints are the most susceptible to strains. The L4–L5 and L5–S1 areas sustain the most intense load and motion, resulting in the most common strain injuries. The most likely coupling patterns, such as axial rotation with lateral bending and lateral bending with flexion–extension, result in load-bearing strain injuries. Lifting weights can also contribute to lumbar strain. Both coupling patterns and lifting weights can create temporary instability, leading to soft tissue injury in the area around the spine.

Treatment for an acute lumbar strain

Treatment for an acute lumbar strain begins with cold therapy to decrease localized tissue inflammation and bed rest for up to 48 hours. Manipulation of the affected area should be avoided. Recent studies indicate that some activity may increase functional recovery. However, sports activities with weight lifting and extreme range of motion at the spine are not recommended while pain is present. Physical therapy is key to promote proper body mechanics through education, thereby decreasing further stress to the injured lumbar area during activities of daily living and through the use of electrical stimulation with ice application. This typically results in decreased pain and inflammation. To decrease muscle spasms, a lumbosacral corset may be prescribed, which can be discontinued when the spasms resolve. Finally, medication treatment includes the use of oral nonsteroidal anti-inflammatory drugs and intramuscular injections of muscle relaxants.

Repetitive stress injuries

Repetitive stress injuries (overuse injuries) or cumulative trauma disorders are the result of repetitive tissue demand, causing tissue damage of tendons, ligaments, neural tissue, and soft tissue. These injuries may occur with occupational, recreational, and habitual activities. Stresses placed on tissue over time include contraction, compression, impingement, vibration, tension, and shear, to which most tissues adapt. Mechanical fatigue is felt to lead to this adaptation; however, unless there is adequate time to heal, the tissues can be injured while adapting to the presenting demands. With added insults, the injury rate exceeds the amount of time required for healing and adaptation. It is imperative to assess the onset and frequency of symptoms as well as factors that alleviate or exacerbate the symptoms. Furthermore, the patient may report a history of clicking, popping, rubbing, and vascular phenomena.

Treatment for repetitive stress injuries

Conservative treatment for repetitive stress injuries, or overuse syndrome, includes medication treatment, physical therapy, and occupational therapy. Taking into consideration a patient's comorbidities, such as diabetes, repetitive stress injuries may be exacerbated by conservative treatment with medications and injections or by surgical procedures. Although rest and avoidance of activity that exacerbates an injury are important, maintenance of the proper range of motion in a nonpainful way is equally important. Therefore, increased complex treatment is necessary. Physical therapy is a vital piece of conservative treatment because of the following: (1) it delivers patient education with psychosocial benefits; (2) it provides supervision of movement of the injured area and a home exercise program; (3) it provides various treatment modalities, such as heat/cold application, iontophoresis, ultrasound or phonophoresis, and transcutaneous electrical nerve stimulation; and (4) it helps to prevent kinesophobia, or sick behaviors, as a result of a fear of ongoing tissue damage with movement.

Treatment for a chronic subdural hematoma

Following assessment of the size, age, and location of a chronic subdural hematoma (SDH), as well as the overall neurological condition of the patient, treatment is planned. With a near-normal neurological presentation, diagnostic imaging may reveal an expanding chronic SDH that warrants neurosurgery. Surgery may be necessary when the SDH produces a significant mass effect, which is confirmed with diagnostic imaging, and when the SDH is symptomatic. It is worth noting that emergency surgery does not always provide a more favorable outcome than urgently scheduled surgery. Once a patient is considered a surgical candidate, the neurosurgeon must determine the appropriate surgical technique. Two burr holes are typically placed on each side of the head for drainage, thus allowing conversion to a craniotomy, if necessary. A closed drainage system may remain in place postoperatively for up to 72 hours. Another technique involves drainage through a twist-drill craniotomy, such as with a subdural evacuating port system.

Treatment for an acute subdural hematoma

Following assessment of the size, age, and location of an acute subdural hematoma (SDH), as well as the overall neurological condition of the patient, treatment is planned. Patients reporting with neurologic signs, including changes in mental status, such as lethargy or a focal neurologic deficit, are further evaluated with computed tomography scanning. With findings that the SDH is thicker than 5 mm, in addition to the neurologic symptoms, surgical evacuation via craniotomy is typically indicated. Occasionally, removal of the bone plate or flap, or a craniectomy, is necessary with increased intracranial pressure. Apart from the patient's Glasgow Coma Scale, surgical evacuation is necessary with an SDH thickness greater than 10 mm or a midline shift greater than 5 mm. If there is an underlying brain injury or complex medical issues, especially in an older patient, a poor outcome may result, even if the hematoma is successfully removed.

Treatment for a muscle contusion

Proper treatment for a muscle contusion helps to decrease hemorrhage and inflammation and control pain. Most health care professionals do not recommend heat during the initial 24–48 hours of injury. Rather, the limb should be immobilized and treated with rest, ice, compression, and elevation for 24 hours, following minor contusions, and for 48 hours, following moderate-to-severe contusions. After 48 hours, re-evaluation determines if additional rehabilitation is necessary; instructions to avoid subsequent trauma to the injured muscle are given at this time. Occupational therapy is necessary to educate the patient regarding the activities of daily living while using appropriate durable medical equipment, such as crutches, if a limb has to be immobilized. Surgical intervention is unnecessary with the sole presence of a contusion, apart from the confirmation of compartment syndrome, which would then indicate emergency surgery. If there is radiographic confirmation of myositis ossificans, orthopedic consultation is needed.

Treatment for vertebral compression fractures

Conservative therapy is the first recommended treatment for a vertebral compression fracture. This includes pain medication, supplements of calcium and vitamin D, external bracing, and rest. Spinal fracture pain significantly improves within a few days to weeks; however, residual pain remains during the healing process. Importantly, rest for only a short period is recommended to eliminate the chance of bone loss with extensive inactivity. Surgical intervention may be indicated for repair of a fracture with persistent pain. For painful, nonhealing spine fractures from osteoporosis or tumors, vertebroplasty is beneficial. Both procedures eliminate or decrease the pain that results from vertebral compression fractures. Occasionally, spinal fusion surgery is indicated with significant vertebral height loss. Contraindications for vertebroplasty include unrelated pain; extensive fractures, involving surrounding structures; or the presence of an infection; it is important to treat an infection before surgical intervention.

Treatment of an unruptured intracranial aneurysm

Controversy exists regarding the treatment of an unruptured intracranial aneurysm. The International Study of Unruptured Intracranial Aneurysms reported a low risk of rupture among patients with no history of subarachnoid hemorrhage. Ongoing treatment guidelines take into consideration the patient's age, history, and the size of the aneurysm. In addition, certain factors, such as a history of cigarette smoking, a family history of aneurysms, polycystic kidney disease, and a diagnosis of systemic lupus erythematosus, can increase the risk of rupture. The surgeon must also consider the morbidity and mortality rates associated with endovascular or surgical intervention, such as silent thromboembolic events or the risk of hemorrhage, respectively, versus the psychological morbidity that the patient may experience while living with an unruptured aneurysm. However, infectious aneurysms, which may resolve with antibiotic therapy, are known to be friable; thus, avoiding surgical intervention because of the risk of hemorrhage is the standard of care.

Surgical treatment of a cavernous angioma

Most cavernous angiomas do not require surgical treatment; however, when indicated, the approach is determined by the location of the tumor. Generally, these tumors are located within the intraocular space, between the optic nerve and the extraocular muscles. The surgical procedure, hemangioma extirpation, typically includes the following steps: (1) an orbitotomy is performed laterally, medially, or anteriorly, depending on the tumor location; (2) all vessels are identified and cauterized with a bipolar cautery; and (3) general blunt dissection of the encapsulated lesion is completed for en-bloc removal. Alternatively, a cryoprobe extirpation can reduce capsular rupture and bleeding; however, this could result in potentially frozen adjacent orbital structures. Additional modalities used for tumor removal include a carbon dioxide laser, a Nd:YAG laser, or Gamma Knife surgery. Finally, neurosurgical or otolaryngologic consultation is recommended should the cavernous hemangioma demonstrate an intracranial component or extend outside the orbit to the facial structures.

Endovascular intervention for carotid dissection

Despite anticoagulant therapy, carotid dissection can lead to stenosis, occlusion, or pseudoaneurysm formation. When a patient is a poor candidate for medical therapy, endovascular intervention in the form of a stent-supported angioplasty may be a viable option; it is both safe and effective in restoring the integrity of the vessel lumen, resulting in a good clinical outcome. Stents can provide the centrifugal force required to allow apposition of a dissected segment to the wall of the vessel, thereby resolving the stenosis and obliterating the false lumen. Stents can also serve as a scaffold, providing mechanical support, for resultant coil embolization of wide-necked pseudoaneurysms related to dissection. This can all be achieved through the procedure, percutaneous stent angioplasty. Medical research shows that endovascular intervention can be beneficial for high-risk patients (i.e., patients with a hemodynamically significant lesion from severe stenosis or a contralateral occlusion, when anticoagulation therapy has failed or is contraindicated).

Stroke care delivered in primary and secondary stroke centers

Two types of stroke centers have been established, based on the recommendations from the Brain Attack Coalition: primary stroke centers (PSCs) and secondary stroke centers (CSCs). The PSCs provide the timely administration of stroke-specific therapy, such as tissue plasminogen activator and general care of the patient with an uncomplicated stroke. In addition to the care provided by the PSCs, the CSCs provide care to patients with hemorrhagic stroke or intracranial hemorrhage and for all patients in need of an intensive care unit. Emergent evaluation by the emergency medical services technicians and the emergency department (e.g., "stroke codes" or "stroke activations") includes vital sign monitoring, laboratory testing, noncontrast computed tomography scanning, and neurologic consultation as well as prompt transport to a PSC or CSC. Facilities with stroke teams in place routinely administer thrombolytics, which result in decreased mortality rates among stroke victims. A stroke system can ensure the timely identification, transport, treatment, and rehabilitation of patients who have experienced a stroke.

Carpal tunnel syndrome

Carpal tunnel syndrome results when the median nerve, which extends through the carpal tunnel of the wrist, is compressed within this space by the tendons or blood vessels that also run along the tunnel. Termed entrapment neuropathy, tendon swelling or inflammation compresses the median nerve and causes discomfort and pain in the hand that may extend up to elbow. The patient may also have difficulty grasping or pinching. In chronic carpal tunnel syndrome, which is observed most frequently, dull, aching pain accompanies progressive sensory and motor dysfunction. The thenar muscle of the thumb may atrophy. Acute carpal tunnel syndrome is rare, and symptoms include severe, sharp pain, hand or wrist swelling, and diminished finger movement. Tasks and occupations that involve highly repetitive or forceful hand motions contribute to development of carpal tunnel syndrome, particularly in younger patients. Other predisposing factors include rheumatoid disease, tenosynovitis, pregnancy, diabetes mellitus, and trauma.

Symptoms of carpal tunnel syndrome may occur sporadically, later becoming more persistent and severe. Debilitating pain usually occurs before motor impairment, but both interfere with normal function. To prevent this condition, take frequent breaks from tasks requiring prolonged or repetitive movements, maintain proper body alignment, and make the environment amenable to this goal (ergonomic design of occupational space). Splinting in a neutral position during repetitive activities and at night, shaking the hand or letting the arm hang may relieve pain. Pain management may also include nonsteroidal anti-inflammatory drugs. Surgical options include open carpal tunnel release, in which an incision is made to expose the carpal ligament and decompress the median nerve. This may be done endoscopically as well, using a smaller incision. The palmar surface takes longer to heal and wound care is important. In addition to post-surgical splinting, use of the hand should be limited, and it should be elevated if swollen. The patient should be trained in care of the wound and splint usage, as well as exercises to prevent stiffness and increase function.

GCS

The Glasgow coma scale (GCS) is commonly used to classify patient level of consciousness, and is particularly suited to assess comatose patients and those in the acute stages of injury. The scale ranges from 3 to 15, with 15 indicating full alertness. Scores between 13 and 15 indicate mild injury, from 9 to 12 indicates moderate injury, and a score less than 8 indicates severe brain injury. To administer the GCS, a series of stimuli are applied to gauge eye opening, motor, and verbal ability, and the response noted. Auditory stimuli are first used: questions are asked and simple commands given with a normal voice, louder vocalization is used if necessary. If patient is responsive, mental status can be assessed based on responses to specific instructions. If patient is unresponsive to auditory cues, tactile stimulation is applied. Begin with gentle shaking or touching, if no response is observed more pressure or pinching is applied to the upper chest or upper back. Responses include bodily or limb withdrawal, or actively pushing away the stimulus or examiner.

LOC

Level of consciousness (LOC) is a major indicator of neurological change, and should be closely monitored in traumatic injury, stroke, and postoperative patients. Consciousness refers to both alertness and cognitive function. The Glasgow coma scale is most commonly used to numerically rank LOC, but qualitative descriptions are also useful. Fully conscious patients are awake and oriented. They comprehend and respond to instructions. Confused patients are disoriented and may have memory deficits. Lethargic patients demonstrate some confusion and slowed responsiveness. Patients in obtundation require stimulation for arousal, can follow commands with continuous stimulation, are able to respond verbally but use few words, and appear drowsy. Stupor is characterized by lack of spontaneous movement or verbalization, and minimal responsiveness. Patients in coma are unarousable and have the eyes closed. Coma can be divided into three levels based on responses to painful stimuli; whereas complete unresponsiveness corresponds with deep coma, in light coma purposeful withdrawal from painful stimuli is noted and brainstem reflexes are intact.

Secondary cellular injury

Primary injury induces damaging secondary processes including ischemia, hypoxia, and secondary axotomy, which activate additional cellular reactions that further perpetuate the injury. Injurious cellular cascades include excitotoxicity, which begins with the release of high concentrations of the excitatory neurotransmitters glutamate and aspartate from axotomized or degenerating neurons. Excessive activation of their receptors leads to abnormal influx of calcium ions, which activate intracellular biochemical signaling cascades that lead to cell death. An influx of sodium ions also carries water into the cell, causing swelling. Blood and damaged cellular components such as neuron membranes leads to free radical production. Free oxygen radicals continue to damage proteins and cell and organelle membranes. Ischemia, or lack of blood supply, disrupts cellular metabolism leading to excitotoxicity and generation of free radicals.

Disc herniation

Herniation of the nucleus pulposus, or rupture of the inner segment of the intervertebral disc through its outer covering (annulus fibrosis), is usually caused by trauma from lifting heavy objects or falling. It usually occurs in the lumbar or cervical regions, and men are affected more often than women. Intervertebral disc herniation is accompanied by severe acute and chronic back pain, as well as pain in the buttock and leg. Pain and other paresthesias occur due to spinal nerve root irritation caused by the protruding disk or herniated nucleus pulposus. Patients exhibit compensatory postures and gait adjustments, accompanied by spasms of the paravertebral muscles. Patients may have some weakness in the leg or foot, but pain often prevents assessment. MRI or CT scan is necessary to confirm diagnosis.

A herniated disc is associated with a certain syndrome of symptoms depending on the level of the injury. Lumbar level herniation typically occurs at L4-L5 or L5-S1, and sometimes L3-L4. With the more common L4-L5 herniation, pain is felt in the hip, groin, side of the thigh and calf, top surface of the foot, and the first three toes. Paresthesias may be felt in the leg or between the toes. Foot drop may be observed, and walking on the heels is difficult. With L5-S1, pain is generally more posterior and lateralized. It is felt in the gluteus, back of the thigh and calf all the way down the leg to the lateral outer surface of the foot. Paresthesias may be perceived in the calf, heel, or foot. Ankle jerk reflex is affected.

Primary herniated disc treatment is aimed at giving the injured area opportunity to heal and preventing further injury. Addressing these points also helps to reduce pain. Initial management typically takes place in the home, and includes lifestyle modifications such as decreased activity and possibly bed rest for up to four days, to avoid stress on the spine from bearing weight or twisting.

Use of a firm mattress can help maintain alignment and hot or cold application to painful areas can control pain. Analgesics, anti-inflammatories, and muscle relaxants also provide pain relief and are conducive to healing. Use pain scales to monitor the response to treatment. Encourage mobility as appropriate: teach range-of-motion exercises, provide assistance or supervise use of assistive devices. Surgery may be considered for patients who do not improve with conservative treatment within 3 months. There are several surgical options, ranging from removal of impinging disc or vertebral tissue to grafting vertebrae together to stabilize the spine.

Cervical strain

Otherwise known as whiplash, strain to the cervical region is very common. It is generally caused by motor vehicle accidents, during falls, or from repetitive malalignment such as holding a phone with the shoulder. The strain may only involve ligaments and muscles of the neck, but vertebral compression may also occur. Pain or stiffness, inflammation, and muscle spasm may be observed, and anti-inflammatory analgesics are the main treatments. It is important to rule out other injuries of the cervical spine, such as spinal cord root compression or vertebral fracture. Abnormal sensation, strength, or reflexes in the arms may indicate nerve root compression.

<u>Treatment for cervical strain injury</u>
With proper recommended treatment, such as rest, ice, and physical therapy, followed by a home exercise program, rapid and full recovery can be accomplished following a cervical strain injury. Following cervical collar placement at the scene of an accident, and once cleared from spinal injury, ice and medications are initiated. Medical studies do not support the use of soft collars over early mobilization and medication. Medications include analgesics to control pain (e.g., acetaminophen), nonsteroidal anti-inflammatory drugs to control pain and decrease inflammation, and muscle relaxants to reduce pain associated with muscle contracture and to aid rest and physical therapy. Typically, a rehabilitation or occupational specialist can provide follow-up for occasional long-term medical management. However, the primary care provider is very valuable in the overall management of care.

The spinal axis components

Interconnected bony, nerve, and soft tissues make up the spinal axis. Vertebral bones form a muscle-bearing flexible column surrounding and protecting the spinal cord. Thirty-three vertebrae make up the spine. The uppermost seven are cervical; these allow movement in multiple directions and thus are vulnerable to certain injuries. The next twelve vertebrae are thoracic. These fix the ribs, and thus are relatively stable. The next five vertebrae are lumbar. The 5 sacral vertebrae are fused together, as are the 4 coccygeal vertebrae. The vertebrae are held in position relative to each other by ligaments. Posterior ligament/soft tissue integrity is especially important for spine stability. The intervertebral discs sit between vertebral bodies and function to absorb stress on vertebral joints. The spinal cord passes through the protective channel formed by the vertebral arches. The functional relationships and interconnected anatomy of each of these components means that injury to any component compromises the integrity of nearby structures and increases susceptibility to further complications.

Spinal cord injury

Impairment syndromes following spinal cord injury depend on the level, cross-sectional location (central, lateral, anterior, peripheral), and completeness of lesioning. Damage to the center of the spinal cord (usually due to edema) causes more upper extremity than lower deficits. Anterior lesions cause loss of pain and temperature sensation. Unilateral cord damage causes ipsilateral paralysis and loss of touch sensation, and contralateral loss of pain and temperature sensation. Bowel and bladder control are affected at all transectional levels, except they may be spared with lesioning below L4. Motor and sensory impairment occur at roughly matched levels. Lesions from C1 to C4 impair both voluntary and involuntary respiration. Cervical lesions are also associated with quadriplegia (may be below the neck, shoulders, or upper arms). Thoracic lesions cause loss of voluntary respiration and paraplegia (may be below mid chest or waist). Lumbar lesions also cause paraplegia affecting most of the legs and pelvis, or the lower legs to feet. L4 to S5 lesions lead to segmental motor control of lower body joints.

All trauma patients should initially be treated as though they have a spinal cord injury. Once damage is verified, special attention should be paid to blood pressure, respiration, temperature control, and complications due to immobility and impaired sensation. The level of spinal transection can be inferred from the superior extent of symptoms, as they occur inferior to the lesion level. Symptoms include skeletal muscle paralysis and deficits in sensation of pain, the viscera, and proprioception. Spinal reflexes and the ability to perspire are also compromised. Respiratory function may be impaired with a high-level lesion. Lack of bowel and bladder control accompanies lesions at almost all spinal levels. Incomplete lesions may spare some of these functions, but spinal shock may acutely eliminate all neurological function below the lesion. Spinal shock is also associated with lowered body temperature (35.5 to 36.6° C, 96 to 98° F). Loss of sympathetic input (neurogenic shock) causes hypotension together with bradycardia.

Traumatic spinal cord injury is likely to go through several levels of management: prehospital, emergency department, intensive care, and possibly surgical. Goals of prehospital management care are to make an initial assessment of spinal and vertebral integrity, stabilize the head and neck to prevent further injury and provide for safe transport to the emergency department. Accident history and mode of transport are noted. Further assessment and stabilization of airway, breathing, and circulation are prime concerns, followed by neurological examination. Ventilator and oxygen support may be required. Spinal cord trauma patients will often have additional injuries, and thorough examination is required to discover and treat them. Spinal cord patients may be candidates for administration of the steroid methylprednisolone. If so, dosing should begin within 3 to 8 hours of injury. Monitoring of ventilation, blood volume, and cardiac function continues in the intensive care unit.

Surgical treatments for spinal cord injury include decompression laminectomy, spinal realignment, and spinal fusing for stabilization. Immobilization is a main tool for nonsurgical management. Various bracing options exist for thoracic and lumbar immobilization. Cervical injuries can be managed with halo skeletal traction. This system maintains alignment. The halo is anchored to the cranium with pins and also fixed to supports connected to a vest. Monitoring traction equipment assures its safe and effective use. Immobilized patients require extensive monitoring and assistance. Respiration or ventilation, circulation, and bowel and bladder status are primary concerns. Traction and immobilization increase the risk of infection and skin breakdown. Range of motion exercises, proper alignment, and frequent repositioning help to minimize discomfort. Adequate fluid and nutritional intake should be encouraged. Emotional support and information about the injury, recovery, and educational/supportive resources should also be provided.

Peripheral nerve trauma

Injury to peripheral nerves may disrupt neuron function without transection (neuropraxia), or damage nervous and connective tissue. Contusion is associated with neuropraxia. If the surrounding connective tissue remains intact (axonotmesis), damaged peripheral nerves may regenerate. If both neuronal and connective tissues are injured, however, surgery is required for recovery. Traumatic laceration, stretch injury, avulsion or tearing, and electrical or thermal energy are all mechanisms of peripheral nerve injury. Symptoms of peripheral nerve trauma include paralysis and loss of sensation in the innervated area, absent or weak deep tendon reflexes, decreased muscle tone and muscle atrophy with time. Transitory spontaneous muscle contractions called fibrillations may be detected with EMG, and multi-muscle fasciculations may also be observed. Transection of sympathetic nerves causes anhidrosis and warm, dry skin.

Patient considerations in the management of peripheral nerve injury include pain and/or paresthesia, and paresis/paralysis. Surgery may address the primary nerve problem. Establishing a baseline of neurological function of the affected limb is useful for monitoring progress. Initial and subsequent assessments should include motor and muscle function, including range of motion, observing for tremors, fibrillations and fasciculations. Assessment of pain, temperature, and pain sensation as well as paresthesia experience should be included. Sensory impairment increases susceptibility to local injury. Additional observations that are indicative of circulatory status or autonomic tone include the color, temperature, and texture of the skin of the affected limb. If immobilization is prescribed, be sure the splint or cast does not compromise blood supply. A secondary sling or pillow support can also provide proper alignment. Supervise or limit ambulation and other activities as ordered. If the favored hand is impaired, accommodations for handedness may help the patient act independently.

Traumatic cerebral injury

Traumatic cerebral injuries are classified as focal, diffuse, or penetrating (usually gunshot), depending on the mode and extent of damage. Cerebral contusions, lacerations, and intracranial hemorrhage are focal injuries. Contusions are cerebral damage that leaves the arachnoid intact. Movement of the brain within the skull causes contusions as intracranial ridges impact the brain, skull fracture with inward displacement can also bruise the brain. Contusions can lead to edema, increased intracranial pressure, mass effect, and herniation. In lacerations, the meninges are torn, along with the cerebral surface. Diffuse injuries include concussion and diffuse axonal injury (DAI). The temporary neurological dysfunction that characterizes concussion occurs with acceleration-deceleration. Mild concussion may cause headache, confusion, or gait disturbances, but in contrast to classic concussion, does not cause loss of consciousness or memory disturbances. Shearing forces cause microscopic axonal and blood vessel tearing along susceptible junctions, leading to DAI.

The variety of brain injuries caused by trauma requires a range of treatments. Noncontrast CT scans are useful for identifying (or ruling out) blood accumulation associated with hemorrhage and hematoma, as well as cerebral edema and anoxia. Small hematomas may reabsorb, but larger hematomas, intraventricular and subarachnoid hemorrhages may require surgery. Surgery may not improve the outcome in intracerebral hemorrhage, reinforcing the importance of supportive care in this case. Penetrating gunshot wounds are generally addressed surgically to remove bone and bullet fragments and evacuate hematomas. Diffuse axonal injury is associated with unconsciousness, but trauma is sometimes not evident at the resolution of a CT scan. Increased intracranial pressure is an issue with each of these conditions. Observation is generally the approach to concussion. Information concerning neurological signs to watch for and instructions for if deterioration occurs should be provided. Contusions and lacerations of the skin require wound care, and skull fractures may necessitate reconstructive surgery.

Initial management of patients with severe traumatic brain injury follows the same principles as for spinal cord injury. Primary concerns are airway patency, respiration, circulation, and level of consciousness. Emergency department care is focused on stabilization; measures also minimize secondary injury. Monitoring intracranial pressure, oxygen supply, and additional systemic problems continues in the intensive care unit. Ventriculostomy is useful to drain cerebral spinal fluid and lower intracranial pressure. Drug treatments should take into account potential effects on cerebral blood flow and oxygen metabolism, as well as intracranial pressure. Sedation can reduce complications from agitation, ventilator asynchrony, and elevated oxygen demand. Analgesics, anticonvulsants, and the osmotic diuretic mannitol further prevent complications associated with pain, seizure, and cerebral edema, respectively. Euvolemia maintained with hypertonic saline regulates intracranial pressure and blood pressure. Stool softeners to prevent constipation further control risk for elevated intracranial pressure.

Cerebrovascular

Cavernous angioma

A cavernous angioma is defined as an abnormal arrangement of vein-like structures with little blood flow within the brain and the spinal cord. It may also be referred to as a cavernoma or cavernous hemangioma. The cavernous angioma presents with symptoms when it begins to bleed, collecting blood around the cavernous malformation, thereby irritating the brain tissue and creating a mass. The mass, in turn, applies pressure on the brain, which may affect bodily functions, such as movement, vision, speech, or sensation. Symptoms may include weakness, numbness, problems with vision or speech, difficulty swallowing or moving the eyes, and problems with balance and coordination. A cavernous angioma of the brain stem, with any mass or amount of fluid, can compress the vital nerves of respiration, gag reflex, heartbeat regulation, temperature regulation, heat and pain sensation, hiccupping, eye movement, swallowing, walking, speech, and control of facial muscles.

Treatment for a stable cavernous angioma
Treatment for a stable cavernous angioma or malformation includes monitoring with magnetic resonance imaging or computed tomography scans every 2 years and administration of antiseizure medication in the presence of seizures. Should the angioma be causing symptoms or growing rapidly, surgical removal of the entire cavernous angioma may be necessary. If any part of the angioma remains, it may begin growing again. A recent nonoperative option is stereotactic radiosurgery, which is indicated for nonaccessible angiomas or bleeding angiomas. Stereotactic radiosurgery delivers precisely aimed, high-dose radiation with three-dimensional computer images for guidance. No general anesthesia or incision is required with radiosurgery; therefore, the patient is allowed to go home the same day. Occasionally, subsequent radiosurgery treatments are indicated. Factors affecting treatment options include age, location, and size of the angioma, presence of bleeding, the growth rate of the angioma, and the presence of symptoms.

Carotid artery dissection

Carotid artery dissection manifests in the presence of an arterial wall hematoma, resulting in a tear that leads to dissection, thereby narrowing the lumen. This dissection can occur spontaneously or be the result of an injury, including trauma or an invasive endovascular manipulation, also referred to as secondary carotid artery dissection. Other examples of associated trauma may result from motor vehicle accidents, such as a whiplash injury; chiropractic manipulation; severe coughing; and intimal tearing after carotid artery catheterization. Spontaneous dissection typically occurs in patients with connective tissue disorders, including Ehlers-Danlos syndrome (type IV); Marfan syndrome; inflammation, such as vasculitis; and fibromuscular dysplasia. Although patients may be asymptomatic, progression to symptoms typically occurs within days or weeks to include tinnitus, pulse awareness, a transient ischemic attack, or a major stroke. In addition, headache, neck pain, and Horner syndrome may precede a cerebral stroke.

Treatment for carotid dissection
During spontaneous carotid dissection, the extracranial portion of the internal carotid artery is typically involved, due to carotid artery compression and stretching against the cervical vertebrae. Less common is intracranial carotid dissection, which is associated with subarachnoid hemorrhage and death. Recommended treatment includes a combination or sole application of medical therapy,

surgical intervention, and endovascular management. With the progression or recurrence of neurologic symptoms, despite maximum medical therapy, surgical intervention may be warranted; however, the risk for increased morbidity looms. Certain situations warrant the use of endovascular intervention, such as: (1) when anticoagulation therapy is not adequate on its own, (2) when the patient is not a surgical candidate, or (3) when the distal dissection is too difficult to access. One such endovascular intervention involves stenting and coil application. This procedure has been shown to keep patients free of recurrent or new ischemic symptoms for approximately 43 months.

Thrombotic ischemic stroke

Thrombotic ischemic stroke is defined as a blocked artery in the brain. Atherosclerosis causes narrowing of the neck and head arteries. Blood cells may collect and clot within these narrowed arteries. When damaged or diseased cerebral arteries are blocked by a blood clot, a thrombotic stroke (i.e., cerebral thrombosis, cerebral infarction) occurs; thrombotic strokes are responsible for 50% of all reported strokes. According to the location of the blockage, a thrombotic ischemic stroke can be divided into large-vessel and small-vessel thromboses. Large-vessel thrombosis involves blockage to the large carotid or middle cerebral arteries. Small-vessel thrombosis involves small deep arteries that penetrate the brain, producing a lacunar stroke. Thrombotic stroke symptoms vary, based on the location that is affected. Symptoms may include headache, dizziness, confusion, one-sided weakness or paralysis, sudden numbness, sudden changes in vision, difficulty walking, incoordination of the arms and hands, and slurred or impaired speech.

Treatment for thrombotic ischemic stroke

Thrombolytic therapy, such as intravenous recombinant tissue-type plasminogen activator, or rt-PA, has been found to be an efficacious treatment for thrombotic ischemic stroke when administered 3–4.5 hours following the onset of stroke symptoms. Factors to consider when deciding on treatment include the pathophysiology, clinical presentation, and the overall evaluation of the patient; it is also important to consider the overall scope of patient care, including supportive care, treatment of neurologic complications, antiplatelet therapy, glycemic control, blood pressure control, and hyperthermia prevention. Delay in seeking care for stroke symptoms, such as when the patient is unable to call for help or when the stroke occurs during sleep, averages the time from symptom onset to presentation to the emergency department at 4–24 hours. Establishing the time of symptom onset is critical to preserve the area of oligemia, by reducing the duration of ischemia; this is done by restoring blood flow to the compromised area.

Hemorrhagic stroke

Approximately 20% of stroke victims are given a diagnosis of hemorrhagic stroke, resulting from sudden bleeding into or next to the brain. The remaining 80% of stroke victims suffer ischemic strokes. Symptoms of a hemorrhagic stroke include an alarming, sudden, severe headache; nausea; vomiting; neck stiffness; and loss of physical or mental capacity. There are three types of hemorrhagic stroke: (1) intracerebral hemorrhage, which occurs in the brain and accounts for most hemorrhagic strokes; (2) intraventricular hemorrhage, with bleeding in the deep fluid-filled spaces; and (3) subarachnoid hemorrhage, with bleeding between the brain and the membrane covering it. Hemorrhage affecting the brain and the surrounding areas is very serious and potentially life-threatening. Many times, the hemorrhage ceases within the first hour after onset. However, if the bleeding continues, the structure of the brain becomes compressed, and the patient dies.

<u>Treatment for hemorrhagic stroke</u>
When considering the treatment of hemorrhagic stroke, the cause of the stroke must be determined, such as hypertension, anticoagulant medication usage, head trauma, or blood vessel malformation. In addition to monitoring, medical treatment includes controlling blood pressure, discontinuing medications known to increase bleeding, administering blood-clotting factors, and controlling the measured pressure within the brain. Surgical treatment may be necessary to stop the bleeding, either within the first 48–72 hours or 1–2 weeks later to allow for the stabilization of the patient. Another intervention includes aneurysm clipping to prevent re-bleeding. A less invasive intervention than aneurysm clipping is coil embolization, which blocks blood flow into the aneurysm and prevents re-rupture. If the hemorrhage is due to an arteriovenous malformation, treatment may involve surgery, radiosurgery, or embolization. Finally, a decompressive craniotomy may be considered if there is increased life-threatening pressure in the brain from the blood clot.

Intracerebral hemorrhage

An intracerebral hemorrhage involves rapid bleeding into the brain and accounts for most of the hemorrhagic strokes. Unlike an ischemic stroke, an intracerebral hemorrhage presents with a steady worsening of initial symptoms as blood accumulates; however, similar to an ischemic stroke, there is sudden numbness or weakness along one side or part of the body, dysphasia, difficulty in understanding language, sudden confusion, and visual impairment in one eye or in half of the visual field. Minutes following the onset of an intracerebral hemorrhage, the person may experience a headache, nausea, or vomiting. The size and location of the bleeding may determine the degree of impairment. For example, weakness in one side of the body may be the result of hemorrhage in the deep structures of the hemisphere on the opposite side. In contrast, visual disturbances and numbness may result on the same side.

<u>Treatment for intracerebral hemorrhage</u>
Medical treatment for intracerebral hemorrhage involves the identification of an underlying coagulopathy or a hemostatic abnormality. For patients with severe coagulation factor deficiency or severe thrombocytopenia, appropriate factor replacement therapy or platelets are administered, respectively. If the patient's international normalized ratio (INR) is elevated because of oral anticoagulant use, warfarin should be withheld and vitamin K–dependent factors and intravenous vitamin K should be administered to correct the INR. In addition, intermittent pneumatic compression and elastic stockings should be used for the prevention of venous thromboembolism. Once the bleeding stops, low-dose, low-molecular-weight heparin or unfractionated heparin may be administered subcutaneously for the prevention of venous thromboembolism, especially in patients with decreased mobility after 1–4 days. Platelet transfusions may be considered when the patient has a history of antiplatelet use; however, this is still considered investigational.

Intraventricular hemorrhage

Intraventricular hemorrhage (IVH) is a result of bleeding into the ventricles or the cerebrospinal fluid-filled areas inside the brain. The source of bleeding may be near or inside the wall that surrounds either ventricle. When this occurs, it may spare healthy brain tissue. This type of hemorrhage is common in infants with a very low birth weight of less than 1,500 g (i.e., 3 lbs, 4 oz). Because the premature blood vessels are fragile and not fully developed, there is a direct correlation between prematurity (with births occurring before 30 weeks' gestation) and the size of the infant with the risk of IVH: the smaller and more premature the infant, the higher the risk of IVH. Risk factors for IVH, in addition to prematurity, include respiratory distress syndrome and hypertension. Although uncommon, IVH can also occur in full-term infants.

<u>Intervention for periventricular hemorrhage–intraventricular hemorrhage</u>
Periventricular hemorrhage–intraventricular hemorrhage (PVH-IVH), involving the periventricular white matter, or motor tracts, is a central nervous system (CNS) lesion that is associated with long-term disability, which affects infants born prematurely. As there is significant morbidity and mortality linked to PVH-IVH, medical care involves supportive care that may be associated with the development of the neonate, such as overall cardiovascular, respiratory, and neurological system care and support. This includes ventilator support, as well as the correction of hypotension, acidosis, and anemia. In the past, serial lumbar punctures were used to treat posthemorrhagic hydrocephalus; however, spontaneous resolution of the hydrocephalus has been shown to occur weeks after onset of the PVH-IVH. Medication therapy with acetazolamide decreases cerebrospinal fluid production, which would otherwise lead to hydrocephalus. Ventriculostomy is used to manage the hydrocephalus while waiting for the proven surgical procedure of ventriculoperitoneal shunting.

Ischemic stroke

Most strokes are ischemic, occurring due to blockade of blood circulation. Narrowing of blood vessel space due to plaque accumulation on vessel walls limits perfusion, as does occlusion caused by circulating thrombi (blood clots) or emboli. Sources of emboli include atherosclerotic plaques, air, fat, and bacterial masses that move through the circulatory system. When circulating thrombi or other emboli become trapped and prevent blood flow, ischemia results. Most ischemic strokes are thrombotic. Ischemia that leads to cell death is termed an infarct. The area of damaged but viable tissue that surrounds an infarcted region is the called the penumbra.

<u>Treatment for ischemic stroke</u>
The time frame from the onset of ischemic stroke symptoms to emergency room presentation can vary from 4–24 hours; thus, it is imperative that care providers are knowledgeable about preventing treatment delays. It is important to assess the length of time during which the patient and the caregivers did not recognize the symptoms of a stroke. Establishing this time frame is imperative when considering whether thrombolytic therapy would be beneficial. Research is underway to determine the best strategies to block the ischemic cascade, thereby preserving the area of oligemia, reducing the ischemia duration, and restoring blood flow to the compromised area. The effects of ischemia can be mitigated by restoring blood flow quickly, thereby rescuing the penumbra cells before irreversible damage takes place, through recanalization strategies, such as intra-arterial approaches and the administration of intravenous recombinant tissue-type plasminogen activator.

Cardiogenic embolic stroke

Origins of emboli that may occlude brain blood vessels and lead to ischemic stroke include substances of coronary origin. So-called cardiogenic embolic strokes result when fragmented plaques from the heart or coronary vessels become dislodged and travel, usually through the left middle cerebral artery, to the brain and become trapped, preventing blood flow to specified vascular territories. Cardiogenic emboli form during atrial fibrillation, myocardial infarction, and congestive heart failure. Other conditions that contribute to cardiogenic emboli formation include atherosclerosis, valvular disease, patent foramen ovale, and atrial septal aneurysm.

Lacunar stroke

Lacunar strokes are caused by ischemia of small, deep arteries. Degeneration of infarcted tissue leaves a characteristic cavity, or lacuna, typically less than 0.5 mm in size. Lacunae are found most often in the basal ganglia, thalamus, internal capsule and pons. Although the infarcted area is small, deficits may be substantial depending on the functional role of the region of damage. The pathology of lacunar stroke differs from large artery ischemia. Lipohyalinosis leads to arterial inelasticity and thickening of the vessel wall, eventually causing thrombosis. Hypertension is the primary risk factor for small artery ischemia.

Treatment for lacunar ischemic stroke

The treatment for lacunar ischemic stroke includes thrombolytic therapy, secondary prevention, carotid endarterectomy, and stroke prevention. In the acute phase of treatment, the National Institute of Neurological Disorders and Stroke trial recommends the intravenous (IV) administration of tissue plasminogen activator with the onset of symptoms of lacunar syndromes secondary to ischemic infarction. Additionally, acute treatment with 160–300 mg of aspirin within 48 hours of symptom onset proved beneficial, as reported by the International Stroke Trial and the Chinese Acute Stroke Trial. The North American Symptomatic Carotid Endarterectomy trial reported beneficial results with lacunar stroke patients with significant carotid stenosis over 50%. Ultimately, health care providers argue that the control of vascular risk factors, such as hypertension, is the best way to prevent lacunar infarctions. Antihypertensive and antiplatelet agents have proven effective in secondary stroke prevention, while anticoagulants have not.

TIA

Transient ischemic attack (TIA) is a "mini" stroke, causing temporary deficits that clear within 24 hours. Carotid TIA is associated with lateralized symptoms such as monocular blindness, contralateral numbness of the face or limbs. Cognition, language, and behavior may also be affected. Vertebrobasilar TIA symptoms include dysarthria, vertigo, dizziness, ataxia, diplopia, and motor and sensory deficits. Acute care may include antiplatelets or anticoagulants. 40% of patients have TIA before a large-vessel stroke, and thus TIA is a major risk factor for ischemia. If TIA is considered a warning, risk modification can prevent development of more serious infarction. Modifiable risk factors include hypertension, smoking, and diabetes.

Internal carotid artery ischemia

There are four cerebral arteries. Two of these, the internal carotid arteries, form the anterior circulation supplying the brain. From the common carotid bifurcation, internal carotid arteries branch into the ophthalmic artery, middle cerebral artery, and anterior cerebral artery. Ischemia in these arterial branches leads to differential signs and symptoms. Blockade within the ophthalmic artery, which supplies the eye, may cause monocular blindness or temporary blurred or foggy vision. Ischemia of the middle cerebral artery, which supplies the lateral cerebrum, is most common. Middle cerebral artery occlusion is associated with motor and sensory deficits of the face or limbs on the contralateral side, including hemiplegia and hemianesthesia, as well as aphasia and hemianopsia. The anterior cerebral artery vascularizes the frontal pole and the medial surface of the frontal and parietal lobes. Anterior cerebral artery ischemia leads to hemiparesis.

Vertebral and cerebellar artery ischemia

There are four cerebral arteries. Two of these, the vertebral arteries, form the posterior circulation supplying the brain. The vertebral arteries unite to form the basilar artery, which divides to form the posterior cerebral arteries. The posterior cerebral arteries supply the medial, inferior, and lateral aspects of the temporal and occipital lobes, as well as the cerebellum, brainstem, and spinal cord. The temporal lobe participates in hearing and speech production, and the occipital lobe is involved in vision. Thus, associated symptoms of posterior cerebral artery ischemia include dysarthria, dysphagia, diplopia, and bilateral blindness, as well as sensorimotor deficits and quadriparesis. Cerebellar arteries supply the cerebellum. Cerebellar function is critical for motor coordination, and cerebellar ischemia is associated with ataxia, vertigo, nystagmus, and dizziness.

Hemorrhagic stroke

About fifteen percent of strokes are hemorrhagic. Damage due to both ischemic and hemorrhagic stroke occurs because of interrupted blood supply. Perfusion is impaired in hemorrhagic stroke due to vessel rupture and bleeding. The mortality rate for hemorrhagic stroke is higher than that of ischemic stroke, and hypertension is major risk factor. Hemorrhagic bleeding due to small artery rupture creates a hematoma, which usually continues to expand over the first 24 hours. This process increases intracranial pressure and cerebral edema. Intracerebral hemorrhage is associated with impaired consciousness, headache, nausea, vomiting, and bradycardia. Hemorrhagic stroke may also cause bleeding in the subarachnoid space, usually due to ruptured aneurysm or arteriovenous malformation.

Stroke/TIA prevention

Stroke and TIA, as well as other cardiovascular diseases, share several risk factors. Cigarette smoking, excessive alcohol intake, illicit drug use, physical inactivity, age, family history of stroke, and prior stroke are all risk factors. Generally, conditions that affect blood flow also impact stroke risk. These include hypertension (uncontrolled or greater than 140/90 mm Hg), high cholesterol levels, and heart disease, including atrial fibrillation. Diabetes also impacts vessel patency. Management of these conditions with pharmacological or behavioral modifications in turn impacts stroke risk. Cessation of smoking and illicit drug use, reducing alcohol intake, consistent exercise and healthy diet are all lifestyle changes that contribute to blood pressure, cholesterol, and diabetes management, thereby reducing stroke risk. Pharmacological options also exist for management of blood pressure and cholesterol levels, and antiplatelet and anticoagulant therapies (particularly with atrial fibrillation or after TIA) reduce the contribution of these conditions to development of stroke. Prevention of cerebrovascular events, particularly serious stroke following TIA, should be a primary goal of patient education.

Stroke/TIA nursing interventions

Acute medical and nursing interventions following cerebrovascular events serve to stabilize the patient and prevent secondary damage. These include thrombolytic and anticoagulant therapies, blood pressure management, and glucose management. Additional therapies are targeted to specific neurological deficits. Nursing and caregiver accommodation for sensory deficits may include approaching from the unaffected side. Reminding the patient to use unimpaired modalities to compensate, such as visually checking limb placement or turning the head to make up for partial blindness also help to support self-awareness. Care should be taken to protect sensory-deficient patients from injury. Patients experiencing language/communication deficits may require short, clear sentences, or gestures, to understand instructions. Avoid abstract statements. Cognitive and self-care deficits also require commensurate accommodation such as dividing tasks into short steps or repeated instructions.

Antiplatelet and anticoagulant therapies are used during acute ischemic stroke and TIA to increase perfusion. Patients with hemorrhagic stroke should not receive these therapies due to the increased risk of bleeding. CT scan without contrast is used to determine if stroke is hemorrhagic. If thrombolytic therapy (t-PA) is used, anticoagulants and antiplatelets should not be used for 24 hours. Anticoagulants such as heparin and warfarin are used to prevent clotting and maintain blood flow. Heparin is administered IV, and warfarin is used orally. Monitor and maintain INR between 2 and 3.5 with anticoagulation therapy. Antiplatelets include aspirin, extended release dipyridamole plus aspirin, ticlopidine, clopidogrel. Recommended doses after TIA or ischemic stroke are 50-325 mg of aspirin daily, 200 mg extended release dipyridamole plus 25 mg aspirin, 500 mg ticlopidine, or 75 mg clopidogrel per day. Patients should be monitored for bleeding, changes in intracranial pressure and intracerebral hemorrhage due to increased blood flow.

Cerebrovascular events

Hypertension is a primary risk factor for TIA, ischemic and hemorrhagic stroke, making blood pressure management of concern in prevention of cerebrovascular problems. Antiplatelet and anticoagulation treatments after TIA, and additional thrombolytic treatments for ischemic stroke are designed to increase blood flow and pressure instability and reperfusion injury may result. Blood pressure monitoring is critical during acute care to control for changes in perfusion. Reperfusion may increase cerebral edema, intracerebral pressure and risk of hemorrhage. Blood pressure management is critical to minimize these risks. Cerebral blood flow may also be facilitated with hypervolemic therapy, which induces a slightly elevated, stable pressure. Intensive blood pressure regulation is important for hemorrhagic patients, particularly as it relates to intracerebral pressure, and should be managed pharmacologically to a systolic pressure between 150 and 170 mm Hg, and mean arterial pressure less than 130 mm Hg.

Neuromotor deficits due to stroke include problems with overall motor coordination and mobility, as well as limb paresis. Location and severity of these deficits have acute diagnostic value, and in the long term can greatly affect patient outcome. The upper limbs, often unilaterally, are particularly affected. Hemiparesis impacts patient ability for self-care and other activities of daily living, self-esteem, and ability to readopt a normal lifestyle. Patients may need assistance with turning, appropriate body alignment, and hand support/splinting to maintain functional positioning. Limited mobility also increases risk of deep vein thrombosis. Rehabilitative therapies to promote mobility and fine motor function include encouraging movement as soon as medical stability allows and passive range of motion exercises. Patient/caregiver should be trained in functional accommodations, exercise, and movement practice plans.

Many discharged stroke or TIA patients will continue on antiplatelet and/or anticoagulant drug therapies. These include aspirin, warfarin, clopidogrel, and ticlopidine. Blood pressure medication may also be prescribed. Patients/caregivers should be educated concerning prescribed dosages and expected side effects (particularly for drugs that were not administered during the hospital stay), as well as the necessity for ongoing monitoring of blood clotting and blood pressure. Medications taken prior to the stroke should be reassessed in view of the revised therapeutic plan.

Stroke and dysphagia

Neuromotor deficits due to stroke include difficulty swallowing and impairment of the gag reflex. Coughing or choking may be observed. Related problems include airway clearance, nutritional support, and difficulty communicating (dysarthria). Evaluate swallowing ability and get approval for oral intake before offering food. To prevent aspiration, elevate the head, and, if applicable, provide nourishment to the unaffected side of the mouth. Nasogastric or orogastric intubation may be necessary for suction or nutrition; these measures should be delayed by 24 hours if t-PA is administered. Weight should be monitored to ensure maintenance. Educate patient/caregiver concerning swallowing assessment and feeding accommodations.

Surgical interventions for stroke

There are few surgical options for stroke patients, but interventions associated with stroke include carotid endarterectomy, extra- or intracranial bypass, and hemicraniectomy. Carotid endarterectomy is recommended for patients with a high degree of stenosis (commonly following TIA) for the prevention of serious stroke. Similarly, cranial bypass surgery may also reduce the stroke risk for some patients with severe narrowing of cervical vessels. Hemicraniectomy, in which a piece of skull is removed, is performed to reduce intracranial pressure due to edema, and is most common following intracerebral hemorrhage.

Carotid endarterectomy

Carotid stenosis, or narrowing of the carotid artery commonly due to occlusion by atherosclerotic plaques, reduces blood flow and is a risk factor for stroke. It may be identified following TIA. Carotid endarterectomy (CEA) is a surgical intervention that treats stenosis for the purpose of preventing ischemic stroke. It may be recommended for patients following TIA. Carotid endarterectomy does not benefit patients with less than 50% stenosis, but patients with stenosis greater than 70% show a significant reduction in stroke risk over the next few years. In this procedure, the atherosclerotic plaque is removed from the carotid region of build-up. Associated risks include mobilization of emboli and blood pressure instability due to carotid manipulation. Postoperatively, systolic blood pressure should be maintained at 150 mm Hg. Facilitated blood flow after surgery increases risks associated with hyperperfusion, including intracerebral hemorrhage, but hypotension can contribute to TIA or stroke. Patient autoregulation of blood pressure may be temporarily impaired, and should be managed to between 120 and 130 mm Hg. Seizures and myocardial infarction are also frequently observed after carotid endarterectomy.

Right hemisphere stroke

Right-hemisphere damaged patients may appear distractible and impulsive, or may have a flattened affect. They may demonstrate left side neglect, characterized by inattention to the left side of the body and stimuli in the left visual field, as well as paralysis of the left side. Headache on the right side may be reported. Other features are not right-left specific, but will show contra- ipsilateral predominance dependent on the specific vascular region that was compromised. With right hemisphere damage, these deficits will be patient-left focused: left visual field, motor, and sensory impairments. Some left-handed people (40%) are right hemisphere dominant, and these people may experience the language and communication problems associated with left hemisphere stroke in the rest of the population. Most people, however, will maintain language function with right hemisphere damage.

Left hemisphere stroke

Right-handed and most left-handed people are left-hemisphere dominant. Language comprehension and production functions are concentrated in the left hemisphere, leading to expressive, receptive, or global aphasia and agraphia with damage on this side. Cognitive abilities may be impaired, and behavior may be slow and careful. Headache on the left side may be reported. Other features are not right-left specific, but will show contra- ipsilateral predominance dependent on the specific vascular region that was compromised. With left hemisphere damage, these deficits will be patient-right focused: right visual field, motor, and sensory impairments.

Depression in stroke

Neurological problems due to stroke may include emotional instability and depression. Almost half of stroke patients experience depression, which may improve with pharmacological treatment. Caregiver and patient education emphasizing the emotional impact of stroke, both direct effects of damage on neurological function and secondary effects due to awareness of deficits (such as hemiparesis) and associated grief is important to prepare these parties to understand and address these issues. Loss of inhibition and other personality and cognitive changes in the patient may also impact the caregiver. The patient and caregiver should be made aware of ongoing medical support and available psychiatric resources.

Patient education

Patient and caregiver education during the hospital stay and at discharge are critical to adherence to the prescribed care plan and favorable outcome in the long term. Following stroke, patients and caregivers should have clear instructions for medication usage and understand their purpose. Train as necessary in feeding/elimination protocols and catheter maintenance. A follow-up plan for assessing neurological and hemovascular health should be agreed upon. A physical therapy regimen should be advised, and resources for continued physical rehabilitation made known. Expectations for changes in communication, self-care, and activities of daily living abilities should be discussed. Means of finding and utilizing family and patient support resources should be clear.

Bowel and bladder function

Bladder and bowel function may be compromised after stroke. Control is affected by motor and sensory deficits, as well as level of consciousness. Offering frequent voiding opportunity can help patients re-establish normal function, prevent urinary tract infection, and mitigate need for catheterization. Profiling the urination pattern with a record of intake and output as well as frequency and forcefulness can help with setting a voiding schedule for bladder retraining. A regular elimination routine may also facilitate normal bowel function. Dehydration and immobility contribute to constipation, which can be treated with dietary roughage, laxatives, or suppositories.

Language/communication deficits

Left hemisphere stroke may damage the primary language comprehension and production centers. This may lead to aphasia, or language impairment. There are 3 types of aphasia: expressive, receptive, and global. Expressive, or nonfluent, aphasia is typified by agrammatical speech and occurs with damage to Broca's area of the frontal cortex. Comprehension is generally spared, and patients are often aware of the deficit. In receptive, or fluent, aphasia speech is composed of meaningless arrangements of words and occurs with damage to Wernicke's area of the temporal lobe. Comprehension is also impaired. Global aphasics have deficits in both production and understanding of language. Other communication disorders associated with stroke include alexia and agraphia, or difficulty with comprehension and production of written language. Accommodation for these deficits during care may include use of short, simple sentences and clear directions including gestures if necessary. Support patient attempts at communication. Patients may not understand written instructions. Patient and caregiver education should include information concerning the specific deficit and recommended practices for effective communication with the patient, as well as language therapy options.

Self-care deficits

Stroke patients may have a variety of impairments with regard to self-care. Sensory and motor deficits, including ataxia, apraxia, and hemiparesis, compromise patient ability to dress and handle toiletries and eating utensils. Compensatory behaviors may be utilized and alternate routines devised in conjunction with the caregiver to establish a manageable degree of independence. Disability due to hemiparesis is often long term, and ongoing rehabilitation should encourage use of and provide practice for the deficient side. Patients with right hemisphere damage may also demonstrate unilateral neglect, in which bodily sensory and motor deficits are accompanied by inattention to the left side of the body. The left limbs, side of the face, and stimuli in the left visual field are ignored. Addressing this condition may include regular reminders for the patient to turn their head and attend to a new field of view.

Stroke diagnostics

Outward symptoms of stroke are common to other problems, making patient history and imaging techniques critical diagnostic contributors. Patient history, including hypertension, atrial fibrillation, diabetes, heart disease, smoking, or obesity places a patient at risk for stroke. Physical assessment should include blood pressure measurements, including standing blood pressures, auscultation of the heart, head and neck to document rhythm and possible bruit indicating stenosis, check for retinal emboli, and blood work including clotting evaluation with prothrombin time (PT) and partial thromboplastin time (PTT). Neurological deficits will vary with the territory of compromised vascularization, and electroencephalogram (EEG) may be necessary to rule out seizure. Various imaging techniques can be used to refine the diagnosis. These include computed tomography (CT) to differentiate between ischemic and hemorrhagic stroke, magnetic resonance imaging (MRI) to visualize damaged tissue, and transcranial doppler and cerebral angiography to assess blood flow and degree of stenosis.

Stroke thrombolytic therapy

Tissue plasminogen activator (t-PA) therapy should be administered within 3 hours of stroke symptom onset. t-PA should not be used in hemorrhagic stroke; CT scan may be used to exclude hemorrhage. Patients eligible to receive thrombolytic therapy have not had recent intracranial or other major surgery, head trauma, myocardial infarction, or gastrointestinal or urinary tract hemorrhage and have blood pressure less than 185 mm Hg systolic and 110 mm Hg diastolic. Patient can not be pregnant or lactating, INR must be less than 1.7 with blood glucose between 50 and 400 mg/dl. Recommended t-PA dose is 0.9 mg/kg administered as a 10% bolus over 1-2 minutes, followed by the remaining 90% given by IV over 1 hour. Other anticoagulants or antiplatelets should not be administered until 24 hours after t-PA administration. After t-PA administration, patients should be monitored in an intensive care unit. Blood pressure should continue to be regulated to less than 185 mm Hg systolic and 110 mm Hg diastolic.

Diagnostic imaging

Various imaging techniques can be used to refine the stroke diagnosis. These include computed tomography (CT) to differentiate between ischemic and hemorrhagic stroke, magnetic resonance imaging (MRI) to visualize damaged tissues, and transcranial doppler and cerebral angiography to assess blood flow and degree of stenosis. Computed tomography (CT) scan with contrast is used to visualize infarcted tissue; without contrast CT is used to differentiate between ischemic and hemorrhagic stroke. Lesioned tissue and vascular structures can be visualized with perfusion MRI, and diffusion weighted MRI can show ischemia early. Transcranial doppler is used to assess circulation and stenosis and is useful for evaluating candidacy for carotid endarterectomy. Cerebral angiography gives even more precise information about the degree of stenosis, and together these two tools are used to evaluate candidacy for carotid endarterectomy.

Glucose management

Hyperglycemia correlates with increased infarct size and fluid retention, and increases the risk of hemorrhage during t-PA treatment. Insulin should be administered to manage serum blood glucose levels. Abnormal glucose levels also influence neurological function, and thus may mask other treatment effects. Saline solutions, not glucose, should be used for all IV fluids for at least 24 hours following stroke. Fluid management is critical to stabilize intracranial pressure, blood pressure and reduce the risk of vasospasm. Glucose, osmolality, and electrolyte concentrations must all be taken into consideration, and appropriate fluid administration needs determined.

Respiration

Airway patency may be compromised in stroke patients due to neurological deficits such as dysphagia or low level of consciousness. Patients that are unable to maintain a clear airway may require intubation or suctioning. Precautions should be taken with suctioning to ensure oxygen maintenance during catheter insertion, and intracranial pressure should also be monitored. Blood gas levels should be monitored and maintained with oxygen therapy if necessary. Respiritive asynchrony in ventilated patients may be resolved with pharmacotherapy to ensure optimal ventilation. Tracheostomy may be considered. Positioning patients on the side prevents accumulation of oral secretions and aspiration; patients should be turned every 2 hours. In addition to airway maintenance concerns, aspiration may lead to pneumonia.

Long term disability

There is a high survival rate for ischemic stroke patients, but most will sustain deficits leading to long term disability. Acute care reinstates medical stability and minimizes the degree of infarction, and extended rehabilitative therapy supports the patient's spared neurological functions and re-trains or develops compensatory strategies to make up for remaining deficits. Long term motor function impairments include paralysis and paresis, or weakness, usually on one side of the body. An arm, leg, part of the face, or the entire side of the body may be affected by damage to brain motor areas, leading to problems with such activities as manipulating objects, walking, and swallowing. Language impairments, or aphasias, include long term difficulties with speaking, comprehension, and reading. As with learning any new skill, re-learning after stroke requires repetition and practice. Physical therapists can provide exercises and activities to encourage and develop skilled use of impaired limbs, and speech-language pathologists teach techniques to improve communication and compensate for language deficiencies. Occupational therapists can integrate the patient's abilities into daily routines.

Intracranial pressure

Declined motor and sensory function, headache, vomiting, and decreased level of consciousness are associated with increased intracranial pressure following intracerebral hemorrhage. Changes in these symptoms should be reported immediately. To manage intracranial pressure, the head of the bed should be kept at a 30 degree angle, and cerebral spinal fluid (CSF) may be drained. Color, clarity, and quantity of drainage should be noted. Osmotic diuretics, hypertonic saline, sedatives, barbiturates, or hyperventilation may be ordered, and euvolemia should be maintained. Intracerebral pressure monitoring carries a risk of cerebral spinal fluid infection, particularly in patients monitored for longer than 5 days, those with cerebral spinal fluid leakage, or those with concurrent infections. Infection may be prevented with maintenance of the catheter insertion site and regular changes. Aseptic technique should also be observed in CSF drainage.

Temperature considerations

Cerebral blood flow and metabolic rate are sensitive to changes in body temperature. High temperature is associated with increased damage and poor outcome following stroke, thus, controlling fever is important to optimal care. In contrast, mild hypothermia appears to have protective effects and is associated with improved outcome. Hypothermia reduces cerebral edema and lowers metabolism and oxygen consumption, reducing the production of free-radicals. Antipyretics may be used to control fever and lowering the room temperature or cooling blankets may be used to further decrease body temperature. Cooling should be done slowly to prevent shivering, which increases intracranial pressure.

Glasgow Coma Scale

The Glasgow Coma Scale (GCS) provides a measure of patient alertness based on verbal, motor, and eye opening responsiveness. It uses a scale from 1 to 15, with higher scores corresponding with higher level of consciousness. GCS score is predictive of prognosis in stroke, although it is typically associated with traumatic brain injury patients. It is generally more applicable to hemorrhagic than ischemic patients, due to the more dynamic changes in intracranial pressure. It is used in monitoring stroke patients, as changes in these neurological parameters are correlated with outcome and also indicative of changes in intracranial pressure. Stroke patients with GCS between 3 and 8 may be of such a low level of consciousness to require ventilation and urinary catheterization.

Aneurysm and subarachnoid hemorrhage

Although headache may be reported, aneurysms generally do not produce symptoms until they bleed, making the focus of clinical management hemorrhage rather than the pathological vessel enlargement. Cerebral angiography and CT scans are useful for diagnosing aneurysm and subarachnoid hemorrhage. Monitoring neurological status, and regulating intracranial pressure, cerebral blood flow, and fluid volume are all acute concerns. Drug control of blood pressure and to prevent seizure may be necessary. A variety of surgical interventions exist to clip or seal off ruptured aneurysms, and post-operative pain should be managed. Treatment within 48 hours is advised to limit the risks associated with therapy, particularly rebleeding.

Patients who survive aneurysm rupture or subarachnoid hemorrhage are at increased risk for repeat bleeding, particularly within the first few days following the initial bleed as normal clots break down. Early surgical or endovascular treatment to seal off the rupture is the best defense against rebleeding. Cerebral vasospasm is a concern mainly from 3 to 14 days after hemorrhage. Narrowing of blood vessels limits cerebral blood flow and can lead to ischemia. Neurological deficits, including reduced level of consciousness, paralysis, and aphasia may accompany cerebral vasospasm. Evaluation of clot size and location can be predictive of the likelihood of developing vasospasm, and neurological functions associated with the vascular territory of the affected vessels more carefully monitored. Dehydration and subsequent increased hemoconcentration affect vasospasm development. Subarachnoid hemorrhage also increases risk of seizure, particularly in combination with hypertension.

Subarachnoid hemorrhage, a type of intracerebral hemorrhage, occurs when aneurysmal blood vessel rupture or trauma leads to bleeding in the subarachnoid space. Vascular malformations are also susceptible to hemorrhage. Aneurysm location determines susceptible rupture sites, and they tend to form at artery branch points. Although only about 7% of strokes are attributable to subarachnoid hemorrhage, a third of these events are lethal. The Hunt-Hess classification is used to rate subarachnoid hemorrhage on a scale from 1, asymptomatic, to 5, deep coma. CT scans image the extent and location of hemorrhage, and cerebral angiograms depict aneurysms and malformations. Susceptibility to rebleeding should be considered during acute management.

Cerebrovascular aneurysm

A cerebrovascular aneurysm is defined as a weakened area of a blood vessel, resulting in vessel wall bulging or ballooning, typically at the branch or fork of a blood vessel where it is more vulnerable. A cerebrovascular, or cranial, aneurysm occurs in the brain. Causes of a cerebrovascular aneurysm include hypertension, atherosclerosis, and head trauma, as well as congenital defects. An unruptured cerebrovascular aneurysm may not present with any symptoms but may be detected by a magnetic resonance angiogram or a carotid angiogram. However, the unruptured aneurysm may present with cranial nerve palsy, pupil dilation, double vision, eye pain above and behind the eye, and a localized headache. In contrast, patients with a ruptured cerebrovascular aneurysm may present with a localized headache, nausea, vomiting, a stiff neck, double or blurred vision, photophobia, and loss of sensation. The rupture can be confirmed by computed tomography scan; lumbar puncture, indicating blood in the cerebrospinal fluid; and cerebral angiogram.

Treatment for cerebrovascular aneurysm

Surgical treatment for cerebrovascular aneurysm involves a craniotomy, or surgical opening of the skull, followed by isolating the aneurysm with clips to allow for deflation and using angiography to visualize the aneurysm closure, thereby ensuring normal blood flow. Surgical repair is not possible if the cerebrovascular aneurysm is situated in an unreachable area of the brain or if the risk of surgery is too high. Endovascular techniques may be used, including the use of microcatheters to deliver coils to the aneurysm, thereby occluding the aneurysm from the inside of the vessel. Balloon-assisted coiling delivers a tiny balloon catheter to keep the coil positioned in place. A combination of a stent and coiling provides a scaffold effect for the coiling with a small flexible cylindrical mesh tube. Clinical outcome is dependent on the size and location of the aneurysm, whether it has ruptured, and the patient's age and general health.

Headache classifications

Headache pain in the absence of pathophysiology or lesion is termed a primary headache. These include migraine, tension-type, and cluster headaches. Migraine headaches are of moderate to severe pain and are often prohibitive to daily activities. Certain factors, such as caffeine, tyramine, stress, changes in length of sleep, and hormonal changes are known triggers. Migraines are sometimes preceded or accompanied by auras, or specific neurological symptoms, including bright lines in the visual field, nausea, and light sensitivity. Tension-type headaches are mild to moderate, and may be acute or chronic. Chronic tension-type headaches last at least 15 days a month for at least 6 months. Muscle contraction may contribute to the pain. Cluster headaches are extremely severe and of short duration, but occur at high frequency (up to 8 daily) for several months. Some may be triggered by vasodilating stimuli. Secondary headaches arise due to pain from underlying abnormality or damage, including aneurysm, subarachnoid hemorrhage, meningitis, tumor, increased intracranial pressure, infections or other problems associated with the eyes, ears, sinuses, or teeth.

Headache management

Primary headache pain can be managed pharmacologically, but lifestyle and behavioral modifications can often decrease their frequency. Early intervention can prevent the progression of the migraine course. Acute pain management is likely to include analgesics such as aspirin, acetaminophen, or ibuprofen. If these are not effective, narcotic analgesics or ergots may be used with care.

Arterial vasoconstriction also reduces symptoms. Antiemetics may be necessary with migraine and ergot therapy. A headache record may help guide the patient through identification and reduction of headache triggers by highlighting patterns in timing of occurrence or dietary links. Educating the patient about common triggers as well as conditions associated with headache such as fluid retention, stress, and sleep disturbances will help them control and prevent headache pain. Because secondary headaches accompany physical damage, treatment of the underlying disorder is critical in addition to pain management.

Acute headache

An acute headache presents with localized pain to the head, sometimes radiating behind the ears and eyes and in the upper neck. Typically, a patient is given a benign diagnosis of acute headache, contributing to approximately 2% of emergency room visits. Patient history is key as most patients do not present with any other physical signs, and proper diagnosis is paramount as 5% of patients presenting with a headache may also be experiencing a condition that warrants immediate attention and intervention. These conditions include: meningitis, epidural hematoma, subdural hematoma, subarachnoid hemorrhage, hypertensive encephalopathy, eclampsia/preeclampsia, giant cell arteritis, and acute angle closure glaucoma. To assist with the proper diagnosis and in addition to the patient's medical history, diagnostic clues are valuable, such as the temporal profile, including onset, episode duration, and sleep patterns; precipitating factors; associated symptoms; and family history. Nearly all men and women experience at least one headache a year.

Treatment for an acute headache

Treatment for an acute headache with an unknown etiology is targeted at stopping the headache or preventing the headache from recurring. With a known cause, treatment is aimed at treating the condition. Treatment to stop a moderate-to-severe, occasional tension-type headache may include over-the-counter pain medicine, a type of analgesic. However, a combination of treatments may be required to prevent headaches that impact the patient's activities of daily living. The combination may include the following: (1) analgesics; (2) antidepressants, used to decrease the frequency and duration of tension-type headaches; (3) biofeedback, which is beneficial in controlling how the body reacts to factors, such as pain or stress; and (4) cognitive-behavioral therapy or stress management. Two types of biofeedback include the following: (1) thermal biofeedback, which measures heat and prevents some headaches when used with relaxation; and (2) electromyographic biofeedback, which measures muscle tension and prevents some headaches when used with other treatments.

Chronic daily headache

Headaches that occur for more than 15 days a month are classified as chronic daily headache (CDH). Sometimes, patients suffer from a daily headache for at least 3 months. There are two categories of CDH, based on duration: (1) headaches lasting longer than 4 hours, including chronic or transformed migraine, chronic tension-type headache, new daily persistent headache, and hemicrania continua; and (2) headaches of less than 4 hours duration, including chronic cluster headache, chronic paroxysmal hemicrania, and short-lasting unilateral neuralgiform headache attacks with conjunctival injection and tearing. Approximately 5% of the population seek medical consultation for daily or near-daily headaches. Overuse of pain relief medication is common and can precipitate or sustain the headache frequency pattern. CDH has been shown to evolve from transformed migraine headaches (most common), new onset headaches, and episodic tension-type headaches.

Treatment for chronic daily headache

Treatment for chronic daily headache (CDH) that occurs more than 15 days a month is often aimed at treating the underlying condition or disease felt to be causing the headaches. When the underlying condition or disease is unknown, treatment is aimed at headache prevention. For the chronic, dull, achy, tension headache, treatment includes over-the-counter (OTC) medication, such as aspirin, ibuprofen, and acetaminophen. Throbbing, severe, often one-sided headaches, which worsen with daily activity and are often accompanied by nausea, vomiting, and light/sound sensitivity, may be treated with OTC and prescription medications; rest in a dark, quiet room; cold or hot compresses to the head and neck; limited caffeine; and massage. With the unpredictable onset and quick subsiding of cluster headaches, OTC analgesics are not an effective treatment. However, treatment includes preventive medication, injectable medication, or nasal sprays for quick relief; oxygen; and rocking or pacing to ease the associated restlessness.

Hemifacial spasm

Stimulation of the facial nerve via compression or irritation can lead to involuntary facial movement, which is typically unilateral and occurs in the fifth or sixth decade of life. Tumor, arteriovenous malformation, or stroke may cause this symptom. Twitching may first be apparent in the eyelids, progressing to eye closure and involvement of other facial muscles over time. Alignment and ability to control the mouth may be compromised. Botulinum injections are used to block the errant neuromuscular signal, thus controlling the muscle contraction. If the cause is identified as an impinging tumor or vascular malformation, other interventions may be warranted.

Spinal vasculature

The vertebral arteries, collaterals of which supply the cervical cord, join with the anterior and posterior spinal arteries, which supply the length of the spinal cord. The ventral-running anterior spinal artery and two dorsal posterior spinal arteries are joined by branches of the deep cervical, intercostal, lumbar, and sacral arteries on the way down. Radicular and radiculospinal arteries provide additional blood, as does the artery of Adamkiewicz, which supplies much of the caudal spinal cord. Dural sinuses, including the cavernous sinus, superior sagittal sinus, and transverse sinus, provide cerebral venous drainage, and, in turn, pass through the spinal region and drain into the jugular veins.

NIHSS

In the National Institutes of Health Stroke Scale (NIHSS), scores are given for each of 11 criteria used to grade neurological function in stroke patients. Scores are predictive of stroke severity and outcome. Level of consciousness is first evaluated based on observed alertness. Ability to answer simple questions and follow motor commands is next assessed, followed by oculomotor control and visual function. Symmetry of facial muscle control, arm and leg motor function, and general coordination are evaluated next. Pin prick is used to assess sensory function. Cognitive and language impairments are highlighted when the patient is asked to describe what is happening in a picture, identify a set of objects, and read sentences (included in the scale). Speaking ability is also scored. Lastly, behavior characteristic of neglect, or inattention, is scored. Total score may range from 0 to 42, with higher scores indicating greater impairment. Mildly impaired patients scoring less than 4 generally show satisfactory recovery and should not be administered t-PA, and scores greater than 22 indicate high risk for hemorrhage.

Head of bed positioning

The elevation of the head of the bed is an important detail in maintaining intracranial pressure during acute care following trauma, stroke, or surgery. Flat positioning facilitates cerebral perfusion pressure, but once it is adequate the head is generally raised. Venous drainage is facilitated by 30 degree elevation, thus impacting intracranial pressure. A patient with low blood volume may experience decreased cerebral perfusion pressure if elevated, so maintaining volume is essential. If an elevated patient is to undergo transport or a procedure requiring flat positioning, they should be lowered 15 minutes prior to the procedure to allow time for associated alterations in intracranial pressure to be addressed. Gradual elevation protocols may be prescribed following surgical procedures.

Treatment for an arteriovenous malformation

Treatment for an arteriovenous malformation (AVM) includes four options: (1) conservative management, (2) stereotactic radiosurgery, (3) immobilization, and (4) surgical removal of the AVM. Conservative management is indicated in elderly, high-risk patients with very large or unruptured AVMs, who, following neurovascular consultation, undergo treatment with antiseizure medication. Stereotactic radiosurgery is indicated for small AVMs (less than 3 cm), for deep AVMs, and for poor surgical candidates; it involves delivering one high dose of radiation to the targeted area, resulting in thickened blood vessels and occlusion for 18 months to 2 years. Immobilization involves blocking the abnormal arteries by injecting a glue-like material, to eliminate small AVMs or to shrink the AVM before stereotactic radiosurgery or surgical intervention. Surgical removal is performed following a thorough evaluation of the AVM location, size, formation, and the artery–vein relationship.

Treatment for an arteriovenous fistula

The most successful treatment for an arteriovenous fistula (AVF) involves either surgery or an interventional treatment, such as occlusion coils or a glue-like substance to the feeding vessel. The latter treatment is reserved for an AVF that is located between a small artery and vein, with the result achieved by blocking the abnormal blood vessel connection. Another endovascular procedure involves stereotactic radiosurgery, which aims radiation at the abnormal blood vessel connection. A more recent minimally invasive endovascular technique covers the communication site between the artery and vein with a stent graft that is deployed within the artery. If the AVF is between a medium or large artery and vein, surgical intervention is recommended as occlusion of the artery could be dangerous. Finally, the surgical approach involves disconnecting the arteriovenous fistulous communication, followed by repair of the defect in the artery and vein.

Treatment for a dural arteriovenous fistula

The treatment for a dural arteriovenous fistula (AVF) includes three options to repair the abnormal passageway between the artery; the dura, which covers the brain or spinal cord; and the vein. The first option involves an endovascular procedure that releases a coil or a glue-like substance through a guided catheter to the dural AVF, thereby blocking the abnormal blood vessel connection. The second option, stereotactic radiosurgery, blocks the abnormal connection of the blood vessels with radiation, which is precisely targeted to the abnormal connection. The third option, surgical intervention, involves disconnecting the dural arteriovenous fistulous communication, followed by repair of the defect between the artery and vein. Ongoing research is underway by neurologists and neurosurgeons in an effort to treat dural AVFs effectively and safely, using minimally invasive techniques during surgical intervention. Such research is documented in the National Library of Medicine publications.

Important Terms

Arterio-venous malformation – developmental vascular defect in which capillaries are lacking and arteries and veins interface directly. Most often found in nervous system vasculature, arterio-venous malformations are susceptible to rupture, leading to intracerebral or subarachnoid hemorrhage.
Aphasia - Set of disorders characterized by difficulty producing or understanding language. Aphasias are not caused by motor control deficits.
Apraxia - Neurologically based inability to initiate voluntary or "on-command" movement, although muscle function is normal.
Diplopia - double vision, objects appear doubled due to ocular misalignment; eyes appear crossed or wander.
Dysphagia - difficulty swallowing due to lack of muscular control.
Dysarthria - speaking difficulty characterized by inarticulate, slurred, slow speech; caused by an inability to coordinate the muscles of the mouth.
Expressive aphasia, characteristic of damage to Broca's area, is typified by non-fluent, agrammatical speech. Comprehension is generally spared. Receptive, or fluent, aphasia occurs with damage to Wernicke's area, and is characterized by speech composed of meaningless arrangements of words. Comprehension is also impaired.
Global aphasics have severe deficits in both production and understanding of language, due to extensive damage to multiple language centers.
INR – international normalized ratio; standard for reporting blood clotting status that takes the specific thromboplastin and testing instrument into account so that ratios are comparable everywhere. This international convention makes INR the preferred unit for reporting prothrombin time.

Prothrombin time (PT) – the time it takes for decalcified plasma to clot after the addition of thromboplastin and calcium; laboratory test of the function of a set of clotting factors that is used to monitor warfarin treatment; due to variability in thromboplastin, results are reported in INR units.

Partial thromboplastin time (PTT) – also activated partial thromboplastin time (aPTT); the time it takes for a clot to form after calcium, phospholipid, and a coagulation activator are added to decalcified blood plasma to activate the intrinsic coagulation pathway; laboratory test of the function of clotting factors other than those tested with PT; termed "partial" because of the absence of thromboplastin, or "tissue factor;" used to monitor heparin treatment.

Aneurysm - blood vessel region of excessive expansion that is susceptible to rupture. Etiology varies and includes trauma, infections, and genetic factors. Patients with unruptured aneurysms are typically asymptomatic.

Berry aneurysm – the most common type of aneurysm, aneurysms in this shape classification are typified by a saccular protrusion connected to the blood vessel by a stem.

Fusiform aneurysm – aneurysm designation based on shape; characterized by blood vessel expansion without a defined stem.

Dissecting aneurysm – when injury due to trauma, atherosclerosis, or inflammation separates vessel wall layers and blood flows into this space an elongated bulge forms.

Giant aneurysm – when classified by size, giant aneurysms are those between 25 and 50 mm.

Arterio-venous fistula – vascular malformation in which an abnormal channel, or fistula, connects an artery and vein. Some arterial blood is shunted prematurely to the vein, diminishing flow of oxygenated blood to target areas and adding abnormal stress to the vein due to the higher arterial pressure. This connection may form an aneurysm. Arterio-venous fistula may be congenital, or may form due to improper healing of neighboring blood vessels.

Dural arterial–venous fistula – most common type of spinal cord vascular malformation, a fistula connecting a feeder artery detours blood to spinal veins, leading to venous congestion and hypertension, as well as hypoperfusion of the spinal cord, which leads to spinal cord dysfunction.

Tumors

Brain tumors

The outward signs of brain tumors depend on the tumor location, size, the type of tissue it originated from, whether the tumor is compressive, and what effects it has on intracranial pressure. Generalized symptoms of tumor may include headache, especially a changed headache pattern that worsens in the morning. Nausea, vomiting, and altered level of consciousness may also occur, usually in response to increased intracranial pressure. Seizures are common with brain tumors, especially those that are slow growing. Focal symptoms are specific to the region or structure affected. They may include personality or emotional changes (frontal lobe syndrome), overactive growth (pituitary), or sensory or motor abnormalities.

Brain tumors are most common in adults over age 55 and children under age 15. In children, most tumors are located in the posterior fossa. One-third of childhood brain tumors are astrocytomas. Medulloblastomas and ependymomas (from cells lining the ventricles) are also common. Pilocytic astrocytoma grade I occurs predominantly in children. In grade I tumors, no atypia, mitosis, endothelial proliferation, or necrosis is observed. Tumors caused by genetic and congenital conditions tend to appear earlier in life than other types of neoplasm. These include neurofibromatosis and craniopharyngioma. Medulloblastomas have the potential to metastasize to the spinal cord. Chemotherapy, which prevents cell division, can impair childhood development and growth. Developmental side effects must be considered when determining a tumor treatment plan.

Tumors add abnormal mass within the confined space of the skull. This causes complications due to increased intracranial pressure and possible herniation. Tumors tend to grow radially. If slow, growth is accommodated by soft cerebral tissue until a rigid structure forces a change in shape. Fast-growing tumors are not accommodated and are likely to show earlier signs of increased intracranial pressure. Some neoplasms occur as diffuse infiltrations of cerebral tissue. Tumors also contribute to increased intracranial pressure by exacerbating edema. Compression of blood vessels causes them to leak plasma, and tumor-released factors affect the blood brain barrier, altering fluid distribution. Tumors may directly obstruct cerebral spinal fluid flow, causing hydrocephalus. Increased intracranial pressure can also cause swelling of the optic nerve, or papilledema, which is associated with changes in vision including diplopia and decreased acuity.

Overall objectives of nursing management of brain tumor patients include providing education to allow patients and their families to make informed decisions, administering treatments to address both the primary condition and to ameliorate therapeutic side effects, and increase patient comfort. Patients and their families may experience fear and anxiety, and require assistance dealing with such issues as social isolation and lifestyle adjustment. Referrals to appropriate resources, support groups or counseling options can help them cope. It may also be useful to use a scale to rank quality of life or functional status to evaluate the effectiveness of interventions over time. Administering drugs to relieve headache, nausea, and vomiting help to reduce discomfort. Anticonvulsants reduce seizure activity, but precautions should still be taken to assure patient safety should they have a seizure. Intracranial pressure is a continuous concern with brain tumor, and monitoring level of consciousness can help identify changes in intracranial pressure.

Embryonic brain tumor

When the fetus begins to develop, a tumor originating in the embryonic, or fetal, tissue of the brain and spinal cord of the central nervous system (CNS) may develop. An embryonic brain tumor consists of rapidly growing cells in masses. Most CNS embryonic tumors are malignant; however, some may be benign. The malignant brain tumors grow rapidly, spreading into other brain tissue. There are many tumor types, including ependymoblastoma; medulloblastoma, including classic, desmoplastic/nodular, anaplastic, and large cell; primitive neuroectodermal tumor, including CNS neuroblastoma, CNS ganglioneuroblastoma, medulloepithelioma, and ependymoblastoma; CNS atypical teratoid/rhabdoid tumor; pineoblastoma; and pineal parenchymal tumor of intermediate differentiation. Factors that determine the prognosis and treatment include the age at which the tumor is diagnosed, the type and location of the tumor, whether any metastasis has been detected, certain chromosomal changes, and whether the tumor is recurrent.

Treatment for an embryonic brain tumor

With the diagnosis of a central nervous system embryonic brain tumor in childhood, surgical intervention typically follows. Before surgery, a needle biopsy may be obtained, first by removing a portion of the skull to expose the area of cancerous tissue. Occasionally, a computer-guided needle is used. Subsequently, pathology confirms the presence of cancer cells, using cytogenic analysis, light and electron microscopy, and immunohistochemistry studies. Biopsy confirmation is followed by the removal of as much of the tumor as possible during the same surgical procedure. Research shows that the extent of the surgical resection, which is the favored method of treatment, is directly related to an increased rate of survival. A small study addressing the administration of presurgical chemotherapy to enhance subsequent resection of a reduced-bulk tumor did not suggest a high or improved rate of survival, nor did it demonstrate a decrease in postoperative complications.

Meningeal brain tumors

Abnormal cells that originate in different parts of the brain or spinal cord tissue of an adult can develop into a primary brain tumor. A brain tumor can also result from metastasis from a tumor in another part of the body (metastatic brain tumor). Metastatic brain tumors are more common than primary brain tumors. There are various types of brain tumors, including meningeal brain tumors (meningiomas). These tumors form in the thin tissue layers covering the brain and spinal cord (i.e., the meninges). They are most common in adults and include three grades of tumors. Grade I tumors, which are most common, are prevalent in women; they are benign and slow growing and typically form in the dura mater covering the brain near the skull. Grades II and III are prevalent in men and include rare, malignant, fast-growing tumors that spread within the brain and spinal cord.

Treatment for a meningeal brain tumor

Treatment for a meningeal brain tumor varies, depending on the grade of the tumor. World Health Organization (WHO) grade I meningiomas are typically curable when resected. In cases where the patient has known or suspected residual disease or has a recurrence of the meningioma after surgical resection, surgery and radiation therapy are recommended. With unresectable tumors, radiation therapy without surgical intervention is the recommended treatment. WHO grade II meningiomas, such as atypical, clear cell, and chordoid tumors, and grade III meningiomas, such as anaplastic/malignant, rhabdoid, and papillary tumors, have worse prognoses because surgical resection is performed less commonly and because of an increased proliferative capacity. The standard treatment of choice involves surgical resection plus radiation therapy. Patients with infrequently curable or unresectable brain tumors can participate in clinical trials that evaluate available criteria for treatment.

Capillary hemangioblastoma

A capillary hemangioblastoma, which is classified as WHO grade I, based on World Health Organization criteria, is associated with von Hippel-Lindau (VHL) disease, which is a familial tumor syndrome. The capillary hemangioblastoma occurs sporadically, typically in adults at an average age of 29 years. Capillary hemangioblastomas may develop in various sites of the central nervous system (CNS), such as the cerebellum, the brain stem, and the spinal cord. However, sporadic tumors are found primarily in the cerebellum. Patients with VHL disease may have multiple capillary hemangioblastomas in various CNS sites. The median life expectancy of a patient with VHL disease is 49 years; the capillary hemangioblastoma is the most likely cause of death. Patients with VHL disease should undergo periodic screening with magnetic resonance imaging. Morbidity and mortality for patients with sporadic capillary hemangioblastomas are low, due to advances in microsurgical techniques.

Treatment of a hemangioblastoma

Treatment of a hemangioblastomas involves surgical excision, which is curative, as this type of tumor is benign and noninvasive, unless surgical intervention is contraindicated due to the patient's comorbidities. The main goal of surgical resection is to preserve the surrounding neural tissue, as the tumors are typically well demarcated with a border of separation, and the tumor does not contain any capsule or membrane. In addition, compression of surrounding healthy tissues must be avoided. Preoperative diagnostic studies are prudent to ensure optimal exposure of the tumor, including magnetic resonance imaging, computed tomography scans, and angiography to identify the blood supply of the tumor. Alternative interventions may also be considered, including: (1) endovascular embolization of the solid portion of the tumor to decrease tumor vascularity and the potential blood loss during resection, (2) stereotactic radiosurgery with the use of a linear accelerator or a Gamma Knife for tumor resection, and (3) antiangiogenic treatment.

Pineal parenchymal brain tumor

The pineal gland in the brain produces melatonin, the hormone that controls the sleep–wake cycle. This gland is made up mostly of pineocytes, or parenchymal cells, which is the origin of the pineal parenchymal brain tumor. This tumor is different from astrocytic and germ cell tumors, which are also pineal gland neoplasms. There are three types of pineal brain tumors: (1) pineocytomas (World Health Organization [WHO] grade II), which are slow-growing with variable prognoses, occurring primarily in young adults; (2) pineoblastomas (WHO grade IV), which are rare, primitive embryonal tumors that are highly malignant, rapid-growing, and more likely to spread, often with a grim prognosis as compared to pineocytomas, occurring primarily in children; and (3) pineal parenchymal tumors of intermediate differentiation, which are considered diverse, monomorphous tumors that are difficult to assign a prognosis because of their unpredictable clinical behavior and growth; they occur in all age-groups.

Treatment of a pineal brain tumor

In clinical trials, treatment of a pineal brain tumor with radiotherapy in patients younger than 3 years of age resulted in increased mortality, as well as significant effects on the child's cognitive development. Additional complications may include endocrine and hypothalamic dysfunction, cerebral necrosis, secondary tumorigenesis, and progression of the disease, such as radiation-induced meningiomas. Determining the application of the radiation, such as whole brain radiation versus focal radiation, is dependent on the histology of the tumor. Postoperative resection of low-grade pineocytomas may help to forego radiation therapy as there is no clinical evidence showing that radiotherapy is a beneficial adjuvant. Patients are monitored for any recurrence or progression of the tumor through serial magnetic resonance imaging scans. Attempts to use prophylactic spinal irradiation have not proven to be medically necessary. For the pediatric patient, radiosurgery in place of radiotherapy is recommended to eliminate or reduce the complications associated with radiotherapy.

Drug therapy

Edema and seizures are common to patients with tumors, and most will receive pharmacological treatment for these conditions. Corticosteroids are administered to reduce edema. Swelling underlies many symptoms, particularly those associated with increased intracranial pressure, and bringing it under control can also relieve these problems. A H2 blocker should also be administered with corticosteroids to prevent gastric irritation. Radiation therapy is also associated with increased edema, and these drugs are also administered during that treatment. Anticonvulsants are used to prevent seizures. Phenytoin and carbamazepine are most commonly prescribed. If a patient is undergoing chemotherapy, they should not receive carbamazepine because it contributes to lowered platelet counts (thrombocytopenia).

Surgical treatment

Options for brain tumor treatment include surgery, radiation therapy, and chemotherapy. Patients may be required to choose amongst these options, and many may undergo more than one at different stages of disease progression. MRI or CT scan is generally used to diagnose tumor, but a surgical biopsy may be done to determine tumor histopathology. However, if the tumor composition is heterogeneous, biopsy may not yield an accurate diagnosis: surgical removal eliminates as much tumor as possible, aggressively managing tumors that may have been inaccurately described. Surgery is also useful for "debulking." Removing mass from accessible tumors often relieves mass effect and decreases elevated intracranial pressure. Sometimes tumors can be completely removed, but even with the residual tumor small, further treatments are more effective.

Radiation therapy

Radiation therapy for brain tumors is often used in conjunction with surgery to get rid of remaining malignant tumor or "seed" cells left behind. Radiation increases survival rates and prevents tumor recurrence. Radiation damages DNA, which kills cells. Tumor cells are more sensitive to radiation than normal cells, which allow targeted radiation to destroy cancerous cells without harming normal ones. Depending on tumor histology, location, and patient tolerance, x-rays or gamma rays are administered daily (standard) or smaller doses multiple times per day (hyperfractionation) over 4 to 8 weeks. Other radiotherapies include stereotactic radiosurgery, in which a focused beam of radiation is used on small tumors, or interstitial brachytherapy, in which a radioactive source is implanted directly in the cavity at surgery. Hypoxic tumor cells are relatively resistant to radiation;

cells in the tumor mass core tend to be hypoxic, limiting the effectiveness of radiation against some tumors.

Nursing management is an important part of providing emotional support during radiation therapy. Preparing the patient for each procedure so they know what to expect and answering questions will help to lessen anxiety. Providing information to the family, especially if the patient's mental function is impaired, is also critical. Reassure the patient that once treatment is complete, the side effects will also resolve. Radiation therapy causes sleepiness, hair loss, and skin problems. Radiation dermatitis occurs at the radiation site, causing redness, tanning, and loss of skin cells. This sensitive skin should be protected from irritation and remain free of cream or cosmetics. Do not wash off localization markings. Plan for patient fatigue and schedule around rest periods. Small meals of easily digestible foods are more likely to be eaten. Nausea, vomiting, and diarrhea may be treated with antiemetics and antidiarrheal agents as necessary. Note complete blood counts. Complications associated with infection, fatigue, and bleeding may arise with bone marrow depression.

Chemotherapy

Chemotherapy is often administered in addition to surgery and radiation. Different combinations of treatments are amenable to different types of tumors at different stages of progression. Chemotherapy drugs interfere with cell division and replication. They target tumor cells because they are rapidly dividing. Systemically administered chemotherapy has some limitations for brain tumors because of the blood brain barrier. Most drugs are administered intravenously or orally. Intra-arterial administration, interstitial (directly into surgical cavity) administration, and intrathecal (directly into cerebral spinal fluid) administration are sometimes possible. These techniques deliver therapy more directly with fewer systemic side effects. Nausea, vomiting, and fatigue occur with chemotherapy, as well as anemia (low red blood cell count), leukopenia (low white blood cell count), and thrombocytopenia (low platelet count). Chronic effects include hepatic, neural, and pulmonary toxicity.

As with radiation therapy, nursing management is an important part of nursing management during chemotherapy. Different chemotherapy drugs induce different side effects, but most cause nausea, vomiting, diarrhea, alopecia (hair loss), and bone marrow depression. Bone marrow depression is evident in changes in the complete blood count: anemia, leukopenia, and thrombocytopenia. Additional complications arise from these conditions. Anemia, or low red blood cell count, is associated with extreme fatigue. With decreased white blood cells, or leukopenia, risk for infection rises and extra precautions against infection should be taken. Thrombocytopenia, or low platelets, is evident in increased bruising and bleeding. Regular monitoring of vital signs and observation for drug toxicity is important.

Neurofibromatosis type I

In neurofibromatosis type I, or Von Recklinghausen's disease, multiple neurofibromas are found along peripheral nerves as well as in the skin. This genetic disorder is associated with a mutation on chromosome 17. Skin hyperpigmentation, brown or tan patches, may be apparent at birth, or develop within a few years; tumors and associated problems occur in childhood. Most patients have small tumors in the iris of the eye. Many have tumors along the optic nerve and will have visual disturbances. Neurofibromas in the periphery affect bone, causing disfigurement, including scoliosis. Many of these children also have learning disabilities. Surgery is sometimes possible, depending on the tumor location and degree of nerve and vasculature incorporation. Neurofibromas tend to be resistant to radiation therapy. Associated skeletal problems must be addressed as well.

Neurofibromatosis type II.

Both schwannomas and neurofibromas are derived from Schwann cells of the peripheral nervous system, but neurofibromas also incorporate other cell types. The tumor involved in neurofibromatosis type II is a schwannoma. In this inherited disorder, the slow growing benign tumor is typically found on the vestibulocochlear (acoustic) nerve. This type of tumor is also called an acoustic neuroma. With involvement of the acoustic nerve, auditory and vestibular symptoms arise such as hearing loss, tinnitus, and vertigo. If the tumor spreads beyond the auditory area, function of the facial, trigeminal, glossopharyngeal, and vagus nerves may also be affected. Incorporation of these cranial nerves may cause diminished sense of taste or facial weakness, difficulty chewing, swallowing, or hoarseness. Cerebellar involvement causes incoordination. Small tumors may be surgically removed, but regrowth is possible if the resection is incomplete. Prognosis is generally good, although hearing and facial sensation may be permanently affected.

Meningiomas

Meningiomas are tumors that arise from the meninges. They originate in the arachnoid layer, and are often attached to the dura. Meningiomas can occur either near the brain or spinal cord. Most meningiomas are slow growing and benign, not eliciting any symptoms. They do, however, compress brain and spinal cord tissue, and may block cerebral spinal fluid flow. They can also erode into bone. With faster growing atypical and malignant meningiomas, symptoms are more pronounced. Brain meningiomas tend to be located between the cerebral hemispheres or under the top of the skull, spinal meningiomas are found along the spinal column. Women develop meningiomas more often than men, and even slow growing tumors grow rapidly during pregnancy. Patients with neurofibromatosis are likely to develop meningiomas. Prognosis is good with complete removal, but meningiomas tend to recur if resection is subtotal. Surgery and radiation are most common treatments, chemotherapy is generally not necessary.

Lymphoma and hemangioblastoma

Lymphomas arise from lymphatic cells. This could occur at nodes, but may be at other areas of lymph distribution; could arise anywhere in the brain. Lymphoma is more common in immunocompromised patients, such as organ transplant recipients and AIDS patients. Lymphomas are usually malignant, often recur after treatment, and do occur in children. Hemangioblastomas are derived from capillary endothelial cells and typically occur in the cerebellum. They can occur sporadically or as part of von Hippel-Lindau disease, which is an inherited syndrome in which tumors develop in several other tissues, including the kidneys and adrenal glands. They are typically benign and slow growing. Cerebellar location may produce ataxia or dizziness.

Pituitary tumors

The pituitary is a neuroendocrine gland that secretes various hormones. Tumors of pituitary origin may also secrete these hormones, and tend to do so excessively. Non-secretory tumors cause symptoms due to compression of adjacent nerves, most notably the optic nerve, causing visual disturbances (scotoma, optic atrophy, paresis of extraocular muscles). Secretory tumors also frequently irritate the optic nerve in addition to producing endocrine disorders. The most common secretion is prolactin, which can cause infertility and amenorrhea. Growth hormone oversecretion can cause giantism (before puberty) or acromegaly (after puberty). Prolactin, growth hormone, and cortisol levels are tested in the diagnosis of pituitary tumor. For some patients with prolactin secreting tumors, prolactin inhibition with bromocriptine may provide sufficient symptom control. Prognosis is good with complete surgical resection. Hormone replacement may be necessary after surgery.

Brain and spinal cord metastases

In contrast to primary tumors that derive from cells of the brain, metastatic brain tumors originate elsewhere. They are usually composed of cells that escaped from lung tumors, or sometimes breast, gastrointestinal, or skin tumors and were spread to the brain via the blood. Metastatic brain tumors can occur anywhere. Spinal cord tumors may come from the lungs, breast, prostate, colon, kidneys, or uterus. The location of the primary organ tends to determine the location of the spinal metastasis because invasion occurs through adjacent vertebrae; the thoracic area is most commonly involved. Most brain tumors do not metastasize elsewhere in the body, but medulloblastomas may migrate to the spinal cord. Like primary tumors, metastatic tumors compress neural tissue and precipitate edema. Prognosis is usually dependent on the primary cancer.

Craniopharyngioma

Craniopharyngioma is a congenital tumor arising from Rathke's pouch of the pituitary. It occurs predominantly in children, but is sometimes observed in adults. Like other pituitary tumors, craniopharyngioma affects endocrine function and may compress the optic nerve. Associated symptoms include growth retardation and visual disturbances. Craniopharyngioma also often impinges on the third ventricle, which may hinder cerebral spinal fluid flow and lead to increased intracranial pressure. Signs associated with elevated intracranial pressure may be the first symptoms noted. Prognosis is good with surgical removal and supplementary radiation therapy. Some patients may require hormone replacement after surgery.

Ependymoma

Ependymomas are primary tumors derived from ependymal cells that line the ventricles and spinal canal. They often occur in children and young adults, and are observed more frequently in men. These slow growing tumors can attach to the ventricle wall and grow into the cerebrum. They often occur in the fourth ventricle and obstruct the flow of cerebral spinal fluid. This causes obstructive hydrocephalus and symptoms associated with increased intracranial pressure, such as altered level of consciousness and seizure. Shunting can relieve the pressure. Tumors are not always surgically accessible, but removal is most effective. Most patients receive radiation therapy; chemotherapy is less effective.

Spinal cord tumors

Spinal cord tumors may be "extramedullary," or "intramedullary." Extramedullary tumors are situated outside of the spinal cord. They may be extradural, or outside the spinal dura within the epidural space, or intradural, within the spinal dura (but outside of the spinal cord). Most extradural-extramedullary primary tumors are chordomas or sarcomas; metastatic spinal cord tumors also usually fit this description. Intradural-extramedullary primary tumors include meningiomas and neurofibromas. This category comprises the highest percentage of spinal cord tumors, and these tumors can often be treated by surgical excision alone. Intramedullary tumors, such as gliomas, invade the spinal cord itself. Intramedullary tumors are difficult to remove completely by surgery without compromising neurological function, and so require a combination of treatments.

Spinal cord tumors share many features with brain tumors, as well as spinal cord injuries. Tumor growth elevates pressure in the vertebral column, which may affect blood vessels and cause ischemia, obstruct cerebral spinal fluid flow, compress and irritate spinal nerve roots, or displace the spinal cord. Slow growing and soft tumors tend to be accommodated by nervous tissue, but fast growing or hard tumors compress the cord. Hard tumors can also cause spinal contusions and ischemia as they do not move or change shape with vertebral column movement. As with brain tumors, spinal tumors cause edema. Pain is usually the first symptom. It may be localized to the involved vertebral area of the back, or cause distributed pain throughout the spinal nerve region of innervation. Bowel, bladder, and sexual dysfunction are common. Motor and sensory deficits are dependent on the spinal level of the tumor, and can be diagnostic.

About half of all spinal cord tumors are found in the thoracic region, and metastatic spinal tumors also tend to occur at this level. Spinal tumor symptoms, as with spinal injury symptoms, are dependent on the level of the lesion. Thoracic symptoms include pain in the chest or back and motor and sensory deficits. Motor problems may include spastic paresis. Sensory abnormalities, such as paresthesia, may be useful in determining the lesion level; hyperesthesia is often noted above the tumor level. Bowel, bladder, and sexual dysfunction may accompany thoracic level tumors. A positive Babinski sign, indicative of corticospinal damage, may be observed. The Babinski reflex is elicited by stimulating the plantar surface of the foot, from heel to toes. This causes dorsiflexion and splaying of the toes.

About one third of all spinal cord tumors occur at the cervical level. Spinal tumor symptoms, as with spinal injury symptoms, are dependent on the level of the lesion. At level C4 and above, patients may experience respiratory problems and quadriparesis. Headache, stiff neck, and paresthesias may also occur. Involvement of the cranial nerves may elicit specific signs, such as difficulty speaking or swallowing with impairment of cranial nerves IX and X. Cranial nerve involvement may also appear as atrophy or difficulty using muscles of the shoulder and neck. Below level C4, pain and paresthesia is focused on the shoulders and arms. Arm weakness occurs as well. Surgical access to cervical level tumors is difficult, making it a less favorable treatment option.

Care of patients with spinal cord tumors shares some commonalities with spinal injury patients, brain tumor patients, and postoperative care issues of other spinal patients. As with spinal injury patients, possible instability may call for bracing or immobilization. A cervical collar may prevent complications from high level tumors. High cervical lesions may also affect respiratory function, and appropriate support should be provided. Spinal tumors, like brain tumors, cause edema. In the confined area of the spine, edema obstructs blood flow and may cause ischemia and infarction. Corticosteroids, usually dexamethasone, are used to reverse edema. Patient positioning for wound access and comfort should be considered.

Administering corticosteroids to control edema, providing for spinal column stability and respiratory support are primary concerns. Monitoring and managing pain are also important. Noting the severity, location, and quality of pain, as well as the effect it has on normal activity, is useful to evaluate the effectiveness of pain-relieving measures. Identify and assist the patient in minimizing aggravating factors. Administer prescribed analgesics. Provide for physical comfort with regular repositioning and diligence with proper body alignment. Monitor factors associated with decreased mobility, including muscle strength and gait. Supervise initial use of assistive devices. Coach range-of-motion exercises to maintain flexibility and tone. Check skin integrity. Patients with sensory deficits may need to learn to protect insensitive areas and monitor them visually. Heat can relieve spasticity, but should be used with care over affected areas to prevent burns. Impaired sensation and physical abilities increase the risk of injury.

Treatment for spinal cord tumors is similar to that available for brain tumors. Surgery is used for biopsy and to relieve pressure. Complete excision is frequently possible, and partial resection also reinstates neurological function. For intramedullary tumors, which are infiltrating and often malignant, total excision would compromise neurological function, but decompression can still improve symptoms. Fortunately surgery is often sufficient for intradural-extramedullary tumors, because spinal cord tissue is less tolerant of radiation therapy than the brain. Radiation is important for treatment of intramedullary tumors and metastases. Radiation myelopathy is a complication of radiation therapy with onset later than six months after treatment is complete. Areas innervated by the affected cord show progressive sensory loss and spastic paraplegia. Chemotherapy is effective for lymphomas and some metastatic lung and breast cancers, and may also be used in adult patients with tumors that are not responsive to other therapies.

Baseline assessment and monitoring of spinal cord tumor patients should include pain, motor and sensory function, bowel and bladder function, and respiratory function. Cervical lesions may compromise respiration. Respiratory quality (depth, rhythm, rate of aspiration), chest movement, and breath sounds should be monitored. Use a pain scale to quantify and track changes in pain over time. Note and prevent exacerbating stimuli. Note movement deficits that impact normal activities. Scale muscle strength, observe tone and examine for atrophy. Check range-of-motion, deep tendon reflexes, coordination and gate. Asymmetrical sensitivity to light touch, temperature, and proprioception can be diagnostic. Document the highest level of normal sensory function on either side of the body. Monitor bowel and bladder voiding patterns. Urinary retention increases risk for infection.

Astrocytoma

Astrocytes are a type of glial brain cell that are star-shaped. A glioma arises from glial cells. Astrocytes maintain the health of nerve cells. There are several types of astrocytic tumors, or astrocytomas, including brain-stem gliomas, which form in and widely spread through the brain stem; pineal astrocytic tumors, which form around the pineal gland; pilocytic astrocytomas, which form in the brain or spinal cord; diffuse astrocytomas, which form mostly in the cerebrum; and anaplastic astrocytomas and glioblastomas, which form mostly in the cerebrum. Mixed gliomas are composed of two types of tumor cells, astrocytes and oligodendrocytes, which mostly form in the cerebrum. Brain-stem gliomas occur rarely in adults and are difficult to cure. Pilocytic astrocytomas occur mostly in children and young adults, especially among those with neurofibromatosis. Diffuse astrocytomas occur mostly in young adults, especially among those with Li-Fraumeni syndrome. Anaplastic astrocytomas and glioblastomas are most common in adults.

Treatment for low- and high-grade astrocytomas
76b Treatment for children with low-grade astrocytomas is determined by the location, the stabilization of visual function, and the possibility of improving survival. For example, an isolated optic nerve tumor warrants a better outcome than a lesion that involves the visual pathway or chiasm. Surgical resection is the primary treatment. However, postoperative medical and psychological deficits may present, such as when a tumor is incompletely resected, leading to subsequent resection, chemotherapy, radiation, or a cerebrospinal fluid diversion procedure (e.g., shunt). Further treatment involves chemotherapy to shrink tumors, delaying radiation therapy. Radiation therapy is typically implemented with progressive disease. The treatment of high-grade astrocytomas in children and adults includes surgery, radiation therapy, and chemotherapy. Importantly, early-phase therapeutic trials may be available from the Children's Oncology Group institutions and the Pediatric Brain Tumor Consortium.

Metastatic spinal cord tumor

A metastatic spinal cord tumor is made up of an abnormal mass of tissue around the spinal cord and spinal column, with uncontrolled multiplication of cells that spread from another site to the spine. The spinal cord tumor can be noncancerous (benign) or cancerous (malignant). Anterior or posterior placement of cervical, thoracic, lumbar, and sacral spinal tumors are further categorized into intradural–extramedullary, intramedullary, and extradural. Bone metastasis most commonly spreads to the spinal column. Lung, breast, and prostate cancers are the primary cancers that typically spread to the spine, lung cancer being most common in men and breast cancer most common in women. Gastrointestinal tract lymphoma, melanoma, kidney sarcoma, and thyroid cancers may also metastasize to the spine. Prognosis with treatment is affected by the nature of the primary cancer, the number of lesions, the presence of distant nonskeletal metastases, and the severity of spinal cord compression.

Treatment for a metastatic spinal cord tumor
With a metastatic spinal cord tumor, there is no proven treatment to increase a patient's life expectancy. The best prognosis is related to the patient's functional score, such as ambulation ability and intact sphincter control. A poor prognosis is associated with a loss of sphincter control, which is typically irreversible. Medical intervention goals include pain control and the preservation

of the patient's overall function. Management of conditions associated with metastatic disease include the management of the following: (1) bone pain, associated with bony destruction or pathologic fractures and treated with oral medication or radiation therapy; (2) neuropathic pain, treated with oral medication or topical preparations; (3) structural stability; (4) hypercalcemia, treated with rehydration and medication; (4) psychological problems; and (5) hormonal manipulation, which works to preserve bone mineralization. Procedures not commonly performed include the treatment of sacral pain and bowel and bladder involvement with neurosurgical ablation, such as a rhizotomy, spinothalamic tractotomy, and cordotomy.

<u>Treatment for a low-grade or anaplastic astrocytoma</u>
Generally, the oncology team, consisting of a medical oncologist, radiation oncologist, neurosurgeon, and neurologist, will choose the treatment regimen needed for a low-grade or anaplastic astrocytoma, including surgical intervention, chemotherapy with adjuvant temozolomide, and radiation therapy; there is no accepted standard of treatment. The best regimen is dependent on the young age of the patient, a lack of clear data to support successful treatment, the morbidity caused by the overall treatment regimen, and the indolent nature of the low-grade astrocytoma. A patient with a history of seizures should continue anticonvulsant therapy, as well as laboratory monitoring of the resultant drug levels. Additional recommended medication includes: (1) corticosteroids, such as dexamethasone, to reduce the effects of the tumor mass, and (2) gastrointestinal ulcer prophylaxis to counteract the potential side effects of the corticosteroid.

<u>Treatment for schwannomas</u>
Schwannomas are benign tumors that often regrow after treatment; they generally compress nerve tissue or nerve bundles. Schwann cells are found at junctions where the central nervous system interfaces with the peripheral nervous system. Of the two possible treatment options available, open surgery or stereotactic radiosurgery (SRS), a general rule is not to proceed with SRS or radiation in young patients to avoid brain stem radiation. In addition, it is important to consider the size and location of the schwannoma when choosing the appropriate treatment option. The operative approach consists of a temporal, lateral, presigmoid, or retrosigmoid craniotomy, with zygomatic osteotomy and apical petrosectomy, using stereotactic magnetic resonance imaging guidance. Simultaneous cranial nerve monitoring, maintenance of a lumbar drain for cerebrospinal fluid, and optimal head positioning are necessary for decreasing the need for significant retraction of the temporal lobe.

The treatment of choice for schwannomas involves surgical resection of the tumor from the nerve, which often results in a cure with no recurrence. Factors to consider when recommending treatment, in addition to the child's age, medical history, and overall health, include the extent of the disease, the expected progression of the disease, and the child's overall tolerance to surgical intervention. As open brain surgery does have potential risks, such as brain damage, cerebrospinal fluid leakage, infection, and hemorrhage, robotic radiosurgery is a noninvasive alternative approach. Radiosurgery is reliable, safe, and precise with minimal to no side effects, as well as virtually no recovery time. Multiple sessions of fractional treatment minimize radiation exposure to the surrounding tissues and structures. Furthermore, radiosurgery is performed on an outpatient basis with no anesthesia. Finally, the overall treatment time with radiosurgery is significantly less than with other radiation therapy options.

Other cranial and spinal nerve brain tumors

Cranial and spinal nerve brain tumors are among a spectrum of primary brain tumors arising from the nerves exiting the brain and spinal cord, such as vestibular (acoustic) schwannomas, arising from the inferior vestibular nerve in the internal auditory canal, and neurofibromas. Occasionally, schwannomas are related to neurofibromatosis, a genetic syndrome. These tumors arise from the nerve sheath of cranial and spinal nerves. Often spinal tumor cells are found with abnormal genes; however, medical research has not found a cause for the genetic alterations. Spinal tumor cells can be familial and are represented by the following: (1) neurofibromatosis, (2) noncancerous tumors developing on or near the hearing nerves, in the arachnoid layer of the spinal cord or in glial cells, and (3) von Hippel-Lindau disease, consisting of noncancerous blood vessel tumors found in the retina, brain, and spinal cord as well as kidney and adrenal gland tumors.

Treatment for an oligodendroglioma

When considering the treatment for an oligodendroglioma, it is important to note that these rare, slow-growing tumors, which originate in the cells that cover and protect brain and spinal cord nerve cells, behave similarly to diffuse astrocytomas. Medical studies indicate that the standard treatment involves surgical resection, followed by radiation therapy. However, patients who undergo surgery with radiation therapy demonstrate little difference in overall survival (5.3 years) as compared to patients who do not have radiation (3.4 years). Furthermore, clinical trials help to determine if viable treatment options are beneficial, including those that administer radiation therapy for incompletely resected tumors with or without chemotherapy, with various drugs indicated, such as temozolomide, or a combination of drugs, such as procarbazine, lomustine, and vincristine (PCV) therapy. Patients are closely monitored to determine response rate as well as any recurrence of disease.

Treatment for neurofibromas

Treatment for neurofibromas (i.e., benign tumors of the peripheral nerves) is surgical. The vestibulocochlear nerve is the most commonly affected nerve, whose function is transmitting sound and balancing information from the inner ear to the brain. The neurosurgeon determines the optimal treatment so as to allow the patient to return to normal functioning with the least disruptive path to the brain and critical nerves. With the vestibulocochlear nerve, the surgical approach, called the endoscopic endonasal approach, is preferred to remove the tumor through the nose and nasal cavities, resulting in decreased recovery time, no disfigurement, and no incisions. The surgeon is able to access the tumor without facial or skull incisions. The major deterrent to surgery is that neurofibromas typically are interwoven into the nerve structure; therefore, there is the potential risk of nerve damage.

Treatment for primary central nervous system lymphoma

Treatment for primary central nervous system lymphoma by surgical decompression with partial or total resection of the tumor has not proven beneficial, with a median survival of 1–5 months, because of the diffuse nature of this lymphoma. Radiation therapy has been the standard treatment with a median survival of 1 year. Despite radiation therapy, the disease recurs in 92% of patients. To increase the chance for survival, clinical trials have included preradiation chemotherapy; however, these combined modality trials have not proven successful. This lack of success is thought to result from the neurologic toxic side effects as well as poor penetration of the drugs through the blood–brain barrier. Offering hope, systemic chemotherapy alone, without radiation therapy, has shown rare instances of neurologic toxic side effects. Another study has evaluated the combination of chemotherapy with autologous peripheral stem cell transplantation, which also did not demonstrate neurologic toxic effects.

Treatment for metastatic brain tumors

Treatment for metastatic brain tumors can vary for a single tumor or for more than one tumor that has spread to the brain from another site in the body. Single-tumor treatment typically includes surgical intervention and whole brain radiation therapy afterward. Multiple-tumor treatment includes surgical biopsy, if the primary tumor type is unknown; whole brain radiation therapy with or without stereotactic radiosurgery; and surgical removal of symptomatic tumors. When surgical intervention is the first line of treatment, and the entire visualized tumor is thought to have been removed, the patient may also undergo adjuvant radiation therapy and chemotherapy to kill any remaining cancer cells and to lower the chance of recurrence. Treatment regimens are considered standard for currently used treatment, while other regimens are tested in various clinical trials. The National Cancer Institute accepts patients with metastatic brain tumors for various clinical trials.

Important Terms

Astrocytoma – glioma derived from astrocytes. Astrocytomas are frequently found in the cerebrum, cerebellum, hypothalamus, optic nerve, pons, and also the spinal cord. Low grade astrocytomas tend to occur more often in children.

Chordoma – tumor derived from embryonic notochord cells. Rare; usually found at the base of the spine; invade both bone and soft tissues causing pain.

Dermoid – teratoma; benign cyst; most occur in young adults, found in sacrococcygeal area, associated with spina bifida.

Ependymoma –glioma derived from ependymal cells that line the ventricles. Typically found in the cerebrum, but can also spread to the spine via the cerebral spinal fluid; spinal ependymomas occur more often in men.

Glioma- tumor derived from glial tissue. Glia include astrocytes, oligodendrocytes, and ependymal cells. Gliomas are the most common type of primary brain tumor. Spinal gliomas are usually cervical.

Meningioma – tumor that arise from the meninges; spinal meningiomas occur more often in women.

Neurofibroma – heterogeneous tumor derived from Schwann cells surrounding peripheral nerves; cannot be resected without damage to the underlying nerve; infiltrates surrounding tissues; genetic origin; in the spine most are located above L1.

Neurofibromatosis type I – genetic disorder in which neurofibromas develop on peripheral nerves and also in the skin.

Neurofibromatosis type II – genetic disorder in which a schwannoma develops on the acoustic nerve.

Oligodendroglioma – glioma derived from oligodendrocytes. Found in the cerebrum; tumors are often calcified; seizure is often the first symptom.

Sarcoma – tumor derived from connective tissue or bone; typically extradural.

Immune/Infection

AIDS dementia

HIV is a blood and bodily fluid-borne virus that is transmitted via sexual contact or other fluid exchange, infected blood transfusions or exposure to infected needles, or from mother to baby. Complications of HIV infection can develop into the disease syndrome AIDS; these complications include other infections and development of some cancers. Effects of AIDS with neuroscience relevance include dementia, myelopathy, and distal symmetrical peripheral neuropathy (DSPN). Early neuroscience symptoms of AIDS are consistent with symptoms of increased intracranial pressure and meningitis. AIDS dementia may begin with minor memory loss or difficulty reading. Tremor or motor clumsiness may occur, as well as depressive feelings. Progressive slowing of mental abilities and motor and gait difficulties limit independence. In the final stages of the disease, the patient has no ability to do activities of daily living and requires constant care.

AIDS has effects on the nervous system, including dementia, myelopathy, and distal symmetrical peripheral neuropathy (DSPN). AIDS myelopathy causes weakness of the lower limbs early on. In advanced AIDS, progressive spinal cord damage leads to gait dysfunction, leg weakness and incontinence. DSPN also affects the lower extremities. It is most commonly observed in late HIV. Symptoms include numbness, tingling or pain in the feet and ankles. These sensations progress from the feet up the legs, are amplified by pressure, and interfere with walking. Acetaminophen or non-steroidal anti-inflammatory medications may be used to manage pain due to myelopathy and DSPN.

The goals of AIDS patient care are to prevent injury with a safe environment, manage pain, and minimize complications. Other infections should be monitored. Arrangements for home care include a regimented medication schedule and bowel and bladder management. Routines with structured daily activities are calming and diversive. Throughout the progression of the disease, the environment must be adapted to maintain safety. Medications for HIV and AIDS patients include antiretroviral therapies, drugs to inhibit HIV replication, and nutritional supplements. Antiemetics may be necessary to counter the nauseating effects of high drug doses. In addition, drug toxicity should be monitored. Sedatives or antidepressants may also be used, and care should be taken to dissociate effects of these drugs from symptoms of dementia when assessing mental status.

Bell's palsy

Bell's palsy is a temporary condition in which irritation of the facial nerve causes unilateral facial paralysis. The nerve may be inflamed or compressed; most cases are caused by herpes virus, but some are idiopathic. Patients that are pregnant, or have diabetes, hypertension, or influenza are predisposed to having this condition. Patients generally experience pain behind one ear, followed by ipsilateral facial weakness. Onset of paralysis is acute, with maximum muscle relaxation and lack of voluntary movement within 48 hours. Taste sensitivity and salivation decrease, while hypersensitivity to sound is common. The eye on the affected side may have reduced watering and the blink reflex is absent. Steroids and antiviral agents lessen symptoms and speed recovery. Due to the vulnerability of the affected eye, it should be lubricated and protected with a patch. Evidence of motor function within a week heralds good recovery; most patients recover within a few weeks, although some retain facial weakness.

Guillain-Barré syndrome

Guillain-Barré syndrome is an autoimmune disorder that is brought on by infection. Macrophages attack myelin surrounding nerves throughout the peripheral nervous system, causing muscle weakness and sometimes sensory loss. In more severe cases, demyelination may be accompanied by axonal degeneration. Over hours or days, the patient experiences ascending weakness and paresthesias, as well as loss of deep tendon reflexes. Weakness of the diaphragm affects respiration. Eventually, facial and ocular muscles are affected. Patients also have abnormal blood pressure and heart arrhythmias. Younger age at onset and less severe symptoms are predictive of a good outcome; some patients may have chronic weakness, but most recover within 12 months.

Flushing out the circulation with plasma exchange every other day for 10 to 15 days, and immunoglobulin IV for 3 to 5 days may limit the autoimmune response. Anaphylaxis, fluid overload, and chills should be monitored throughout these procedures. Vital signs and neurological status, as well as progression of weakness and respiratory function should be assessed regularly. Monitor respiratory rate, breath sounds, and arterial blood gases; if the airway is compromised, suction, intubation, and supplemental oxygen may be necessary. Provide pain scales to assess pain levels and the effectiveness of medication in order to optimize management. Some patients may be unable to use verbal responses, although they understand commands. Provide for communication with a pad and pencil, eye blinks, or other system. The patient should be trained in range-of-motion exercises to be done 4 times per day, and also in the safe use of adaptive mobility equipment such as canes or walkers.

The progression of Guillain-Barré syndrome in children is the same as in adults, except children are less able to communicate their symptoms. Pain and discomfort may be expressed as irritation or uncooperativeness. Intravenous immunoglobulin is used in children to confine the autoimmune response. Analgesics including acetaminophen and ibuprofen may be used to manage pain. Age-appropriate pain scales should be used to assess and adjust medication. Although pain may be intermittent, its severity generally warrants continuous treatment. Anticonvulsants may also be useful. Relaxing and distracting activities help children to cope with pain and discomfort. Most children will make full recoveries.

Lyme disease

Lyme disease is caused by a spirochete that is transmitted from ticks to their blood meal host. It is most common in regions and seasons where ticks frequent: the northeast, north central and midwest Unites States, in late spring and summer. To prevent tick bites, wear light colored clothing and long sleeves to better detect and remove ticks, apply repellent, and check thoroughly for ticks after being outdoors. If found on the skin, take care to remove the tick completely. Pets should also be monitored for ticks and vaccinated annually. In the first stage of the disease, a characteristic rash (erythema migrans) expands from the bite site, and headache, fatigue, and flu-like symptoms develop. Over several weeks, headache and neck stiffness continue, and difficulty concentrating, motor incoordination, and cardiac abnormalities develop. After months, arthritis and joint swelling and pain, particularly in the knees, is observed. In the chronic phase, cognitive changes and fatigue predominate. Antibiotics are used to treat patients with Lyme disease. Most recover with no permanent neurological deficits, although some may have chronic fatigue and joint problems.

Neurocysticercosis

Nervous system infection by the encysted larval form of the pig tapeworm Taenia solium is called neurocysticercosis. Ingestion of tapeworm eggs through contaminated water or food leads to this parasitic disease. After the eggs hatch in the gastrointestinal tract, they enter the bloodstream. From there, they migrate into muscle, eye, or brain parenchyma, ventricles, or subarachnoid space. While the parasite is alive within its fluid-filled cyst, hosts are asymptomatic. The tapeworm can remain in this stage for months or years. In the vesicular colloidal stage, the cyst begins to die. A host immune response is activated, and the cyst wall thickens and the fluid becomes cloudy. Patients experience fatigue, abdominal pain, weight loss, and diarrhea. As the cyst continues to dye, the walls are replaced by granulation tissue and the infection enters the granular nodular stage. In the final stage, which can take 3 to 10 or more years to reach, the dead cyst becomes calcified. Patients may be asymptomatic at this time, or experience continued symptoms including seizures and hydrocephalus if the cyst is located in the central nervous system.

Cysticercosis and neurocysticercosis are caused by parasitic infection by the pig tapeworm Taenia solium. Ingestion of tapeworm eggs through contaminated water or food leads to this parasitic disease. Cyst implantation may cause headache and increased intracranial pressure. Increased pressure contributes to nausea, blurred vision and dizziness. Patients may be confused, inattentive, or have balance problems. Seizures, acute pain, and gastrointestinal complications are also common. Symptoms all together or cyst location itself may interfere with mobility. Cysts located obstructively may cause hydrocephalus, and late stage calcification may make this condition chronic.

Tapeworm transmission is rare within the United States, so travel history, or contact with immigrants or other travelers may be informative as to possible sources of infection. When traveling, particularly in developing areas, be aware of food and water sources. Thoroughly cooking pork and avoiding water that may come into contact with human stool prevents transmission of the eggs, as does maintaining hygiene and hand washing standards. These measures also prevent re- or autoinfection. Antiparasitic agents are administered to hasten the death of the cysts; this occurs within 2 to 5 days. Patients with hydrocephalus should have a ventriculoperitoneal shunt implanted prior to antiparasitic treatment. The host immune system responds when the cyst begins to die, and corticosteroids are administered to limit this inflammatory response. Patients should recover without lasting neurological problems or seizures.

CJD

Creutzfeldt-Jakob disease (CJD) is one of several transmissible spongiform encephalopathies (TSEs). TSEs are caused by prions, uniquely misformed proteins that propagate their deleterious shape (and so infect their host) by unknown mechanisms. The normal form of the protein is harmless, but when mutation causes prion-type misfolding (could be sporadic or inherited), or prion-infected animal tissues are ingested (bovine spongiform encephalopathy), CJD develops. CJD originating from an ingested source is termed variant CJD (vCJD). Most cases are sporadic, not familial or transmitted. Prions accumulate and form plaques in nervous tissue, destroying neurons and creating widespread holes. A person may be infected for over 20 years before symptoms appear, but once they do, life expectancy is typically less than one year. Symptoms progress quickly and include dementia (forgetfulness, easily distracted), motor difficulties (myoclonus and incoordination), and seizure.

There is no medical treatment for Creutzfeldt-Jakob disease (CJD). This terminal disease progresses rapidly, and supportive care is most important to assure maximal comfort for the patient, and coping for caregivers. This may include analgesics and anticonvulsants to control seizure and myoclonus. Dementia may overcome patients within six months, rendering them completely dependent for self-care. Providing information about the disease and support resources may help family and caregivers prepare both emotionally and logistically for this rapid decline. In the course of care, it is also prudent to exercise precaution against prion transmission by evaluating CJD history of prospective organ donors and appropriate treatment of surgical or other potentially contaminated instruments.

Brain abscesses

Abscesses are infected regions in which the local immune response also breaks down tissue. Pus, including liquefied tissue, white blood cells, and remains of bacteria or viruses, is surrounded initially by fibroblasts and later by connective tissue. The infections that lead to brain abscess formation usually begin in the ears, sinuses, or mastoid, but they can originate anywhere in the circulation. Abscesses develop in different brain areas, depending on the source of the infection. Location affects neurological symptoms, but many patients will display increased white blood cells, localized headache, confusion, and drowsiness. Seizures may develop. As the abscess enlarges over a few weeks, these symptoms become more severe. Intracranial pressure may increase, causing herniation. Frontal lobe abscesses may correspond with contralateral hemiparesis and language difficulties. Temporal location may cause contralateral facial weakness and visual deficits, and cerebellar abscess is associated with ipsilateral hemiparesis and gaze difficulties.

Recognizing the primary infection, often the ear, sinus, or lung, can help diagnose and treat abscesses. Treating these infections initially also reduces the likelihood of abscess formation. Antimicrobial treatments destroy the source infection. Elevated intracranial pressure may be lethal, as can abscess rupture into the ventricles. Managing pressure as the abscess occupies more volume prevents these problems. Mannitol may be used to control edema. Abscesses may be surgically excised if the surrounding membrane allows, or aspirated and drained. The surrounding area is typically treated with antimicrobials to prevent reinfection and new abscess formation. Patients may retain susceptibility to seizures after the abscess is removed.

Encephalitis

Inflammation of the brain is termed encephalitis. It is usually caused by viruses, but bacteria, fungi, or parasites may also cause cerebral inflammation. Encephalitis is typically accompanied by meningitis. Many viral encephalitis viruses are transmitted by mosquitoes, and thus are more likely to occur in certain geographical regions at specific times of year. The herpes simplex virus, which also causes cold sores, can cause encephalitis. Symptoms commence gradually and include fever, headache, stiff neck, restlessness, drowsiness, abnormal reflexes, nausea, and vomiting. Altered level of consciousness, seizure, and stupor may also occur. Severe encephalitis may lead to edema and hemorrhage, which further elevate intracranial pressure. Cranial hypertension may compromise respiration and cause coma. Although most encephalitis patients will recover with prompt treatment, different viruses are associated with encephalitis of varying severity. Patients may sustain mental deficits, epilepsy, dementia, paresis, deafness, or blindness.

Precautions against mosquito bites, such as wearing long sleeve clothing while in areas where the insect population is dense prevents the transmission of several encephalitis-causing viruses. Management is similar to that of meningitis. Vital and neurological signs should be assessed regularly, along with respiratory function, in order to monitor progress or check deterioration. Drugs may be administered to prevent seizures, control temperature, and manage headache pain. The antiviral acyclovir is effective against herpes simplex encephalitis. Other comfort-promoting measures include maintaining a cool room temperature, lowering the lights (patient may be sensitive to light), and elevating the head of the bed to 30 degrees. If intracranial pressure increases, it requires monitoring and management. Raising the bed side rails and observing the patient frequently will help to assure safety in case of seizure or due to restless movement. Patients with lowered level of consciousness may need assistance with positioning, drainage, and suction, in order to maintain a patent airway.

Meningitis

Meningitis is typically bacterial or viral in origin and affects the arachnoid and pia layers, as well as the subarachnoid space and the cerebral spinal fluid (CSF) within it. Bacteria may spread to the CSF from infected sinuses, mastoids, or other nearby bones, as well as via the circulation from the lungs. Surgery or invasive trauma may also expose the CSF to infecting agents. Bacterial build up initiates events that block the flow of CSF while increasing permeability of the blood-brain barrier, leading to edema and increased intracranial pressure. Young children may exhibit fever, vomiting, and swollen fontanels. In adults, characteristic symptoms include high fever, severe headache, stiff neck, and altered level of consciousness. Disorientation may progress rapidly to stupor and coma. Light sensitivity and seizures are common. Meningococcal meningitis is specifically linked with risk for adrenal hemorrhage and the presence of petechiae, or small hemorrhages, on the skin or conjunctiva.

Meningitis often occurs with encephalitis, and management of both conditions is similar. Regular monitoring of vital signs, neurological signs, and respiratory function is necessary to track changes. Pain, typically headache and backache, should also be rated in order to gauge the effectiveness of analgesic and comfort-promoting measures. Antimicrobial medications should target the bacteria of origin, and be adjusted as diagnostics dictate. Analgesics, antipyretics, and anticonvulsants may be prescribed. Lowering the room temperature can also help control fever. Perspiration in response to elevated temperature may lead to dehydration; fluid replacement may be required. Precautions, such as raising the bed side rails, should be taken to assure a safe environment in case of seizure. Increased intracranial pressure should be monitored and managed by elevating the head of the bed and mannitol. Immobility and disuse should be addressed. Proper body alignment should be maintained, and positions should facilitate oral and nasal drainage.

Viral meningitis

Viral meningitis (aseptic meningitis), inflammation of the meninges covering the brain and spinal cord, is the most common form of meningitis; bacterial meningitis is the second most common form. Viral meningitis presents with 7–10 days of symptoms followed by a complete recovery, provided the patient has a normal immune system. Viral infections (e.g., enteroviruses, coxsackieviruses, echoviruses, mumps, herpesviruses, measles, influenza, arboviruses, lymphocytic choriomeningitis virus) can lead to viral meningitis, mostly occurring in the summer and fall months in the United States. Presenting quickly or over several days, symptoms include a cold with runny nose, diarrhea, vomiting, or other infectious signs and symptoms. Symptoms specific to adults and older children include high fever, severe headache, stiff neck, sensitivity to bright light, nausea, vomiting, lack of appetite, sleepiness, or difficulty waking up. Infants display irritability, poor eating, fever, and difficulty waking up.

Treatment for viral meningitis

As antibiotics are not effective in the treatment for viral meningitis, the administration of analgesics for headache relief and antipyretics to reduce fever, fluid intake, and bed rest are recommended. Many patients recover completely at home within 2 weeks; however, severe cases or immunocompromised patients may require hospitalization. Ultimately, the prevention or reduction of the risk of becoming infected with viruses that can develop into viral meningitis is vital. Therefore, the following measures are recommended: (1) the maintenance of good hygiene practices, as defined by the Centers for Disease Control, such as proper hand washing; prophylactic oral precautions, including covering the mouth when coughing; and cleaning contaminated surfaces; (2) the administration of childhood immunizations, including the measles, mumps, and rubella vaccine and the varicella vaccine; (3) the avoidance of bites from mosquitoes or other insects that may carry disease; and (4) proper house cleaning in a rodent-infested home.

Fungal meningitis

A rare form of meningitis is caused by fungi and parasites; it can be related to certain immunosuppressant drugs (e.g., steroids, anti-tumor necrosis factor medications), but it is not contagious. Unlike bacterial and viral meningitis, fungal meningitis is not transmitted from person to person. Environmental factors that place people at risk include the inhalation of fungal spores, leading to a fungal infection of the spinal cord. For example, inhaling soil contaminated with bird droppings can lead to a *Cryptococcus* infection, and inhalation of bird or bat droppings can lead to a *Histoplasma* infection. Decaying organic matter can lead to a *Blastomyces* infection, and a

Coccidioides infection can be acquired from soil in endemic areas. Many individuals at high risk for acquiring fungal meningitis have preexisting conditions, such as diabetes mellitus, cancer, or an HIV infection. Finally, the fungus, *Candida*, can be acquired in a hospital setting and spread to the spinal cord through blood.

Treatment for fungal meningitis

The recommended treatment for fungal meningitis is medication management, including the following: (1) antifungal medication to kill the fungus and prevent the fungus from returning, (2) antinausea medication for the prevention of vomiting and to calm the stomach, (3) steroids for pain relief and the reduction of redness and swelling, (4) acetaminophen for the reduction of pain and fever, and (5) additional pain medication. Specifically, antifungal medication, such as amphotericin B, is typically administered intravenously, which may be combined with the oral administration of 5-flucytosine. When indicated, administration may be necessary through a catheter placed directly into the ventricles for cerebrospinal fluid administration. Furthermore, a shunt procedure may be indicated for the treatment of resultant hydrocephalus. Later in the treatment course, the oral administration of fluconazole may be effective. If a patient with AIDS recovers from cryptococcal meningitis, preventing the return of this infection is often managed with long-term medication.

Intracranial hypertension

Increased intracranial pressure is associated with a number of neurological and physiological problems, including altered level of consciousness, stroke, seizures, and herniation. Nervous system infection and associated immune responses often cause intracranial pressure to rise. Hydrocephalus, also a feature of infection, may be the cause of increased pressure. Changes in neurological status, including pupillary responsiveness, motor and vision changes may be indicative of increased intracranial pressure. Headache, nausea, vomiting, seizures, and neck stiffness may occur. Noting baseline vital signs is important because alterations in their status may occur with intracranial hypertension. Intracranial pressure can be monitored directly. Management includes administration of osmolar diuretics such as mannitol, and fluids to maintain euvolemia. Elevating the head of the bed facilitates venous drainage. Stool softeners and other precautions against constipation prevent Valsalva's maneuver, which reduces venous flow. Surgical decompression is also possible.

Hydrocephalus

Hydrocephalus, or cerebral spinal fluid accumulation in the ventricles, occurs when production of fluid exceeds absorption or circulation is abnormal. These conditions occur with meningeal infection or cysticercosis. Elevated intracranial pressure may indicate hydrocephalus, particularly in the case of infection. Hydrocephalus causes headache, nausea, vomiting, lethargy, ataxia, and incontinence. A ventriculoperitoneal shunt may be surgically implanted to drain excess fluid from the ventricles to the peritoneum. It is important to monitor neurological status and vital signs with hydrocephalus to track changes both before and after shunt placement. In addition, the shunt itself requires monitoring and care to prevent malfunction and infection.

Obstructive hydrocephalus

When cerebrospinal fluid (CSF) passage is blocked, an abnormal amount of CSF can accumulate in the brain, building up within the ventricle and causing pressure on surrounding brain tissue, which is referred to as obstructive hydrocephalus. Obstructive hydrocephalus is common in the following groups: (1) infants, as a result of a genetic malformation of the spine or following brain hemorrhage, (2) young children, and (3) adults over 60 years of age. The latter population group may develop obstructive hydrocephalus as the result of a brain tumor or cyst, head injury, or an infection, such as meningitis. Symptoms are attributed to increased pressure on the brain and include the following: (1) in infants, vomiting, drowsiness, irritability, constant downward gaze, seizures, and poor appetite; (2) in children, headache, nausea, fever, decreased concentration, and loss of sensory or motor functions with poor coordination and delayed walking and talking; (3) in older children or adults, impaired vision and bladder control.

Treatment for obstructive hydrocephalus

Selecting the appropriate treatment for obstructive hydrocephalus is determined by the severity of the condition and the cause of the obstruction. When temporary obstruction is present with no reportable symptoms, treatment may not be recommended. With symptoms, surgical removal of a tumor or cyst is recommended, unless the location does not warrant removal. In that situation, surgery is performed to redirect the cerebrospinal fluid (CSF) flow and to decrease pressure on the brain as a result of CSF accumulation, often requiring long-term management. Diverting the CSF can be accomplished by two methods: (1) surgical shunt insertion for redirection of the CSF to a body cavity, and (2) ventriculoscopy or endoscopic third ventriculostomy (ETV), to allow the CSF to flow out of the ventricle to be reabsorbed by the brain. Shunt complications include infection, malfunction of the shunt, and obstruction of the shunt's tubing, whereas, the ETV hole may close over time.

Normal pressure hydrocephalus

Hydrocephalus refers to an excessive accumulation of cerebrospinal fluid (CSF). Normal pressure hydrocephalus (NPH) is defined as the absence of papilledema with normal CSF opening pressure; it is considered idiopathic in 50% of patients but is also related to head injury, subarachnoid hemorrhage, meningitis, central nervous system tumors, and a history of congenital hydrocephalus. NPH is most common in the elderly population. It is represented by a gradually progressive array of symptoms, including apraxia (a movement disorder); bradykinesia (decreased spontaneity of movement); a broad-based, shuffling gait; urinary frequency, urgency, and frank incontinence; and dementia, including prominent memory loss and bradyphrenia (slowness in mental processing). The dementia is thought to be reversible. A detailed history, physical examination, and imaging tests (e.g., computed tomography scan, magnetic resonance imaging) are invaluable for diagnosis.

Treatment for normal pressure hydrocephalus

The main treatment for normal pressure hydrocephalus is surgical cerebrospinal fluid (CSF) shunting. Predictive testing is necessary to ensure that patients will benefit surgically. Following a neuropsychological evaluation to determine a baseline, the patient undergoes a timed walking test with gait videotaping and a lumbar puncture to drain approximately 50 mL of CSF. Three hours later, this testing is repeated, and a significant improvement helps to predict whether shunt surgery would be successful. Occasionally, the improvement may not be noticed for 1–2 days. Additional predictive testing techniques include: (1) placement of external lumbar drainage with an indwelling CSF catheter, (2) CSF infusion testing with two lumbar drains placed for infusion and pressure monitoring, and (3) isotope cisternography, involving the injection of a radiolabeled isotope into the CSF space for monitoring. Ultimately, a good response to predictive testing indicates successful ventriculoperitoneal or ventriculoatrial shunting.

MS

Multiple sclerosis (MS) is an autoimmune disease in which the patient's immune system attacks the myelin insulation surrounding neuron axons, causing demyelination. MS affects women twice as often as men, and onset is usually between the ages of 20 and 40 years. Loss of myelin creates focal lesions and plaques, which usually appear in multiple areas. Myelin is essential for normal propagation of neural transmissions, and demyelination leads to delayed or blocked conduction, as well as abnormal crosswalk. Areas most often affected include the optic nerves, brain stem, cerebellum, and spinal cord. Lesions in these areas cause optic neuritis (blurred vision and blind spots, pain with eye movement), diplopia, ataxia, paresis, and paresthesias. Patients may also experience diminished proprioception and perception of temperature, as well as experience sexual dysfunction. In most cases, neurological symptoms are recurrent, but eventually axons as well as myelin are damaged, and disabilities become permanent.

Presentation of multiple sclerosis (MS) follows different patterns of symptom recurrence and courses of deterioration. In relapsing-remitting MS (RRMS), periodic lapses in neurological function last for days or weeks, followed by a period of remission, which may last for weeks or years. No further deterioration is observed between attacks. This pattern typifies the early stage of the disease for the majority of cases. When the pattern associated with RRMS transforms to include neurological decline between relapses, the disease is termed secondary progressive MS. Continuous deterioration, without remission, is observed in this subtype. The pattern in progressive relapsing MS is one of gradual neurological decline from onset, with superimposed periods of more severe symptoms. Primary progressive MS is characterized by continuous deterioration from symptom onset, without remission or attacks, although neurological status may temporarily plateau. Relapses may be triggered by infection, physical or emotional stress, temperature changes (particularly heat, even a hot bath), fatigue, or menstruation.

Although symptom management is currently the mainstay of care, there are three pharmacological options that reduce the occurrence of symptom relapse and the development of new lesions in relapsing-remitting and secondary progressive multiple sclerosis. These drugs are interferon beta 1a and 1b, and glatiramer acetate. All courses of treatment are expensive. Most patients are treated with one of the interferons, but there is not evidence to clinically differentiate between them. Patients receiving one of these treatments may begin to produce neutralizing antibodies, rendering them therapeutically ineffective in the long-term. The corticosteroid anti-inflammatory methylprednisolone may also be administered for acute relapse.

During remissions, life is generally normal, but symptom management is important during relapses. Patient and caregiver education is critical to emotionally prepare and logistically adjust for relapses and progressive disability. Depression is common, and antidepressants may be prescribed. Exercise, especially stretching, helps to control spasticity, movement disorders, and combats fatigue. Botulinum toxin may be used to manage severe spasticity. Gait retraining and assistive devices may help to maintain ambulation. Patients should be prepared with alternate means of avoiding injury, such as using vision to make up for proprioception deficits and to detect other dangers that touch perception may not be sensitive to, such as heat. Protection from temperature change can help to avoid relapse. Urinary problems may be addressed with self-catheterization or anticholinergics.

ALS

Amyotrophic lateral sclerosis (ALS) is a neurodegenerative disease affecting both the upper and lower motor neurons. Progressive destruction of these neurons that normally stimulate the muscles leads to muscle wasting and corresponding loss of function. Upper motor neuron (corticospinal) degeneration results in uncoordinated muscle fiber recruitment evident in spasticity accompanied by weakness. Lower motor neuron (spinal motor neurons, cranial nerves) involvement leads to muscle fasciculations, atrophy, and paralysis. The culmination of degeneration is respiratory paralysis, causing death within three to five years of onset. Cognition and sensation are not affected. Some cases are genetic, but most are sporadic and men are affected more often than women. Clumsiness is first noted, due to muscle weakness and atrophy in the hands. The tongue is also affected, causing dysarthria and dysphagia. Fatigue and cramping occurs later in the lower limbs. Bowel and bladder function are generally spared until late in the progression.

There is no treatment for amyotrophic lateral sclerosis (ALS), but proactive therapy and education can prolong independence and ease lifestyle transitions as the disease progresses. Physical therapy, range-of-motion exercises, and assistive devices can help to retain motor control apart from spasticity and weakness. Likewise, speech and respiratory therapies promote functional control as long as possible. Drugs may be administered for spasticity. Special difficulties arise with the impairment of the muscles involved in speech, swallowing, and respiration. Communication, nutrition intake, and breathing are compromised, and the patient is prone to aspiration. Providing alternate means of communication, adequate nutrition (gastrostomy tube), and ventilator support are all options to consider. Providing information and referrals to additional resources or support groups allows for proactive decision-making about all stages of care. Because the progression of the disease is known, patients and their families should be encouraged to make decisions regarding end-of-life care while they are able to articulate them. Decisions regarding life-sustaining gastrostomy tube placement and mechanical ventilation are particularly important.

Myasthenia gravis (MG)

Myasthenia gravis (MG) is an autoimmune disorder in which immune system antibodies affect the function of acetylcholine receptors at the neuromuscular junction. Acetylcholine is the neurotransmitter released from motor neurons that stimulates muscle contraction, and receptor failure diminishes voluntary muscle control. Women are affected more often than men, and their symptoms begin earlier in life. The progression of MG is sometimes gradual with periods of unchanged function, and sometimes additional muscle groups are quickly involved. MG is characterized by voluntary muscle weakness and rapid fatigue. The extraocular muscles are typically affected first, causing ptosis and diplopia. Facial muscle involvement affects facial expression, and masticator fatigue makes eating difficult. Muscles involved in speech are also affected. Generalized weakness is also noted. Involvement of the diaphragm and intercostal muscles affects respiration.

There is no cure for myasthenia gravis (MG), but treatments are generally effective at managing the symptoms of this formerly fatal disease. Anticholinesterase drugs inhibit cholinesterase, the enzyme that degrades acetylcholine, thereby prolonging the activity of acetylcholine at the neuromuscular junction. Pyridostigmine is most commonly used. Dosing varies between patients, and can be timed to optimize function for certain activities, such as eating. Increased acetylcholine availability also affects transmission at muscarinic receptors, causing gastrointestinal problems, bradycardia, and bronchoconstriction. Atropine can counteract excessively adverse effects. Immunosupression can be achieved in the long term with corticosteroids, or acutely with plasmapheresis or IV immunoglobulin. Thymectomy is highly successful, with or without thymoma, but is contraindicated for children. Patients often have difficulty swallowing and find chewing fatiguing, and so must take care when eating to avoid respiration. Patients should plan for fatigue and develop schedules to accommodate rest periods. Myasthenia crisis occurs when involvement of the respiratory muscles causes dyspnea. Intubation and ventilation may be necessary.

Seizures

Seizures and secondary injury

Patients have seizures in many settings, but neuroscience patients are often at particular risk. Effects of seizure activity may include loss of consciousness, salivation, bowel and bladder incontinence, and apnea, elevating risk of falling and injury, aspiration, and acidosis. Precautions for seizure include maintenance of low bed position with side rails up and suction and oral airway on hand. Stay with the patient throughout the seizure. Guide movements to prevent injury; this may include easing the patient to the floor from a seated position during the seizure or beforehand if a forewarning aura is reported. Place patient on their side to facilitate drainage and suction to prevent aspiration and maintain a patent airway. Observe and document the length of time the seizure lasted, and note details to describe the seizure including types of movement and body parts involved, pupil size, level of consciousness, and whether there was incontinence. Monitor neurological status and vital signs afterward, noting post-seizure behavior including paralysis and whether the patient slept.

Epilepsy

A seizure is a distinct event in which abnormal neural activation, which may be focal or generalized, causes temporary neurological changes, evident in such symptoms as loss of consciousness, abnormal motor patterns, and hallucination. Epilepsy, or seizure disorder, is a condition in which multiple recurrent seizures occur. Ionic balance is fundamental to normal neural function, and conditions that alter this balance predispose neurons to uncontrolled discharge, or excitation. These patterns of electrical overactivity can be observed with an electroencephalogram (EEG). The cause of most seizures is idiopathic, but other causes include brain trauma and illicit drug use, particularly in younger patients, and brain tumor, alcohol withdrawal, and metabolic disorders. In patients with epilepsy, various "triggers" elicit seizure activity. Fatigue, sleep deprivation, hypoglycemia, drinking alcohol, constipation, and hyperventilation are generalized triggers, but some patients are responsive to specific stimuli, such as flashing lights.

Seizure disorder treatment

Patient education and support help them anticipate and cope with lifestyle changes will help in the adjustment to living with the disorder. If an underlying seizure-causing condition, such as a brain tumor, is identified, it can be treated. Identifying and avoiding external triggers can reduce seizure frequency. Antiepileptic drugs are often effective at controlling seizure recurrence, and surgery is also an option for some patients. It is important to identify the specific type of seizure experienced, because some drugs are effective for multiple types of seizures, others are more specific or can exacerbate other forms. Long term compliance may be necessary for seizure control, and the variety of drug options allows for customized therapy to achieve maximal benefit while minimizing side effects. Dosages and effectiveness evaluations should be documented in a drug diary, particularly while changes are made or a new drug added. About one-fifth of patients do not achieve seizure control with antiepileptic drugs. If a unilateral epileptogenic focus is identified, they may be a candidate for surgical excision of the abnormal tissue.

Important Terms

Absence seizure- type of generalized seizure with brief lapse in consciousness.

Generalized seizure- no focal origin, generalized bilateral discharge.

Partial seizure- focal origin, categorized as simple, complex, or may evolve into a secondary generalized seizure. In simple partial seizures, consciousness is intact and symptoms interfere with distinct categories of function such as motor or sensory. In complex partial seizures, consciousness is impaired, and patients display automatisms, or involuntary repetitive motor activity.

Status epilepticus- medical emergency in which seizing occurs continuously or with onset overlapping such that recovery is incomplete between episodes.

Tonic-clonic seizure- most common type of generalized seizure; has distinct course of progression. In the tonic phase, voluntary muscles contract, producing a stiff posture. Contractions become rhythmic and repetitive in the clonic phase, and hyperventilation and profuse salivation occur. In the postictal phase, clonic movements slow and the patient awakens disoriented. Often they will sleep for several hours afterward.

Pseudoseizures

An abnormal electrical discharge from the brain results in epileptic seizures. In contrast, pseudoseizures, or psychogenic nonepileptic seizures (PNES), are felt to arise from emotional or stress-related psychological issues. Often, PNES are misdiagnosed as epileptic seizures because of their resemblance to paroxysmal episodes. A variety of terms describing PNES have been used in the medical literature, such as pseudoseizures, nonepileptic seizures, nonepileptic events, and psychogenic seizures; however, currently the preferred term is PNES. Paroxysmal nonepileptic episodes can be categorized as organic (e.g., syncope, migraine, transient ischemic attacks) or psychogenic. PNES are a type of somatoform disorder and are further categorized as a conversion disorder; they are often involuntary. In the general population, PNES are diagnosed at the same rate as trigeminal neuralgia and multiple sclerosis. Rare instances of feigning, or voluntarily faking a seizure, are seen with malingering and factitious disorder.

Treatment for psychogenic nonepileptic seizures

It is crucial to deliver the correct diagnosis of psychogenic nonepileptic seizures (PNES), or pseudoseizures, to patients and their families, for adequate understanding, which can ultimately affect the outcome of the planned treatment. Many of these patients have previously received a diagnosis of epilepsy; therefore, they are very resistant to the diagnosis of PNES, often exhibiting denial, disbelief, hostility, or anger. Patients and their families will not be compliant with treatment recommendations without an understanding and acceptance of the psychogenic symptoms; therefore, written information is valuable to supplement the information given verbally. Treatment of PNES should ultimately be provided by a mental health professional, as psychogenic symptoms are considered a psychiatric problem. Management can include psychotherapy and medications, aimed at treating the depression or coexisting anxiety. Studies show that cognitive-behavioral therapy reduced the reported seizure activity significantly.

Treatment for complex partial seizures

Treatment for complex partial seizures may include pharmacologic therapy and, occasionally, epilepsy surgery. When determining whether anticonvulsant therapy should be initiated, consideration involves any electroencephalographic abnormalities, the diagnosis of epilepsy, and a physician-to-patient discussion. Monotherapy with one antiepileptic drug (AED) is considered before polytherapy; the drug of choice is based on drug interactions and side effects, with high doses needed for optimal seizure control before initiating a second AED. Common side effects of the AEDs, which are central nervous system depressants, include sedation, dizziness, and cognitive changes. Despite the initiation of two or more AEDs, epilepsy surgery may be considered, including temporal lobectomy, extratemporal resections, corpus callosotomy, hemispherectomy, multiple subpial transsection, and the placement of a vagus nerve stimulator.

Treatment of generalized tonic–clonic seizures

Anticonvulsant therapy with antiepileptic drugs (AEDs) is indicated for the treatment of generalized tonic–clonic seizures (GTCS), otherwise known as grand mal seizures. The AED is prescribed based on the patient's needs and the epilepsy syndrome, in addition to the seizure type. For patients with multiple seizure types, such as GTCS, valproic acid is generally the first choice for an agent. This is based on an unblinded, controlled, randomized study, the Standard Antiepileptic and New Antiepileptic Drug study, which compared the effectiveness of valproate, lamotrigine, and topiramate in treating generalized epilepsy. Newer medications, such as lamotrigine, topiramate, zonisamide, and levetiracetam, have demonstrated better side effect profiles, when compared to older AEDs, such as phenytoin and carbamazepine. The decline in the use of phenobarbital is the result of the reported adverse cognitive effects associated with this drug. The Food and Drug Administration has approved phenobarbital only for the treatment of partial seizures, vagus nerve stimulation, and some GTCS.

Treatment for status epilepticus

Status epilepticus (SE), or an acute prolonged epileptic crisis, can be divided into three groups: (1) an exacerbation of a preexisting seizure disorder, (2) an initial manifestation of a seizure disorder, or (3) an insult apart from a seizure disorder. The most common cause of SE with known epilepsy is a medication change. Aggressive treatment is indicated for generalized tonic–clonic SE and subtle SE, including maintenance of respiratory function and vital signs, which may include intubation. The ABCs of emergency care—(A) attention to airway, (B) breathing, and (C) circulation— are often jeopardized by generalized convulsive SE and are infrequently affected by epilepsy partialis continua. As SE is life-threatening, hospital admission is imperative. Health care professionals must decide between treatment with excessive medication and the possibility of temporary adverse side effects or the possibility of irreversible brain damage or death. In addition, systemic acidosis is typically transient in nature, and medical research suggests that there are inherent antiseizure effects from acidosis.

Developmental/Degenerative

Arnold-Chiari malformation

Also known as Chiari malformation or cerebellomedullary malformation syndrome, this deformity is characterized by an abnormally small posterior fossa and herniation of the cerebellar tonsils. Displaced cerebellum or brain stem may protrude into the spinal column, obstructing flow of cerebral spinal fluid, and brain stem medullary compression may interfere with respiration. Women are affected four times more often than men. Severity of the malformation is used to classify it, with most falling into type I and type II categories. Type I is less severe, and is often not diagnosed until the third or fourth decade of life. Cerebellar tissue is displaced 3 to 5 mm caudal to the foramen magnum, and appears deformed. Type II is usually associated with spina bifida and myelomeningocele, and is often diagnosed in childhood. In type III malformations, cervical meningocele are present at birth and these infants have a poor prognosis.

Cerebral palsy

The term cerebral palsy is used to describe a set of conditions affecting movement control. It is typically diagnosed early in life, and symptoms do not worsen with time. Symptoms include increased muscle tension, which interferes with both fine and gross movement, and sometimes seizure or mental retardation. A variety of factors appear to influence development of the disorder, including maternal infection or trauma, multiple births, smoking, and alcohol exposure. Complications in delivery, such as hypoxia, may also lead to cerebral palsy. Muscle spasticity may be controlled with drugs, such as baclofen, diazepam, and dantrolene. Botulinum toxin is also in clinical trials. Daily stretching throughout the range of motion is important to maintain joint flexibility and prevent muscle rigidity.

Arnold-Chiari malformation

Type I Arnold-Chiari malformation is generally not diagnosed until adulthood and the precipitating symptom is usually headache. Dizziness and unsteadiness are also reported. Bending forward or looking up may worsen all of these symptoms. Neck, back, and sometimes arm pain are common, as are dysphagia, shortness of breath, and hoarseness. The gag reflex may be absent. Vision problems, such as blurred vision, diplopia, or scotoma may occur. In addition to neurological exam, diagnostic MRI is used to visualize the malformation. Surgery to relieve cerebellar pressure may be recommended for symptomatic patients. This surgery involves posterior fossa craniectomy, cervical laminectomy, and duraplasty. Postoperatively, patients will require pain control with antispasmodics and nonsteroidal anti-inflammatory drugs, and antiemetics to ameliorate nausea.

Hydrocephalus

Hydrocephalus refers to both a congenital condition and an acquired syndrome in which cerebral spinal fluid flow or absorption is impaired and ventricular fluid accumulates. It is associated with elevated intracranial pressure, increased cerebral spinal fluid volume, and ventricle dilation. Acquired hydrocephalus occurs secondary to other conditions, such as obstruction of cerebral spinal fluid flow in Arnold-Chiari malformation, subarachnoid or intracranial hemorrhage, infection, tumor, or trauma. Infants will have an enlarged head and prominent scalp veins. They may be lethargic and have poor appetite. Adults experience headache, nausea and vision problems. In older adults, confusion and impaired cognition, motor instability, and urinary incontinence due to hydrocephalus may be falsely attributed to other causes.

Hydrocephalus treatment

Ventriculoperitoneal shunting relieves fluid accumulation. A ventricular catheter connected to a shunt valve that automatically opens at certain pressures to allow draining is surgically implanted. Medication (furosemide and acetazolamide) may be used to temporarily reduce the production of cerebral spinal fluid, thereby controlling volume. Signs of infection should be monitored, as well as cerebral spinal fluid status and catheter sites. Cerebral spinal fluid leakage increases risk of infection. Patients may experience headache, neck or back pain, or intraperitoneal irritation, which should be managed with analgesics. Neurological status and intracranial pressure should be monitored throughout hydrocephalus care. Patient education is important to continued maintenance of the shunt and ability to recognize associated problems such as shunt failure or infection.

Treatment for communicating hydrocephalus

Communicating hydrocephalus, or full communication between the subarachnoid space and the ventricles, is caused by the following mechanisms: (1) defective cerebrospinal fluid (CSF) absorption, (2) venous drainage insufficiency, and (3) CSF overproduction, which is rare. Medication treatment to decrease CSF secretion in the choroid plexus or to increase CSF reabsorption may be effective in delaying surgical intervention. Such is the case with a premature infant and resulting posthemorrhagic hydrocephalus, when normal CSF absorption resumes on its own. If indicated, repeated lumbar punctures are performed with a communicating hydrocephalus, such as with intraventricular hemorrhage. Surgical treatment (i.e., shunting) is often the preferred therapeutic option. Shunting establishes communication between ventricular or lumbar CSF to a drainage cavity, such as the peritoneum, right atrium, or pleura. Alternatives to shunting are recommended before shunting to avoid shunt complications.

Syringomyelia

Syringomyelia is a condition characterized by the presence of longitudinal fluid-filled cysts (syrinx) within the spinal cord. It is usually attributable to Arnold-Chiari malformation, although other posterior fossa pathologies may contribute to its development. Cerebral spinal fluid flow obstruction, spinal cord injury, hemorrhage, infection, injection, spinal dysraphism, and intermedullary tumors may all lead to syringomyelia. Headaches are the most common symptom, along with pain and weakness of the arms and legs due to compression of the spinal cord. In children, scoliosis may develop as the syrinx enlarges. MRI imaging with and without contrast along the spine is used for diagnosis. Syrinx development is most common in the cervical region, and least common in the lumbar spine. Surgical procedures to alleviate symptoms include posterior fossa decompression, tumor removal, and syrinx drainage. Secondary scoliosis is amenable to treatment.

Myelomeningocele

Myelomeningocele is the most severe type of spina bifida. A myelomeningocele is a herniation of the spinal meninges that protrudes beyond the spinal column and involves the spinal cord, causing abnormal deformation and exposure of neural tissue. It is associated with Arnold-Chiari malformation type II. Most myelomeningoceles are found in the lumbro-sacral vertebral arches.

Symptoms include weakness, paralysis, and lack of sensation in the lower body, as well as a lack of bowel and bladder function. It may also contribute to hydrocephalus. Surgery within 24 hours of birth may be ordered to repair the defect, and postoperative care should include temperature monitoring, positioning of the infant to avoid pressure on the back, and precautions against infection.

Spina bifida

Also known as spinal dysraphism, spina bifida is the failure of the neural tube to close completely. Spina bifida defects may be closed, termed occulta, or more severe and open, termed cystica or aperta. Spina bifida aperta allows meningeal sacs to protrude from the spinal column. Meningocele include only the meninges, but myelomeningocele also involve the spinal cord. Herniated sacs are visible in spina bifida aperta. Inability to move the legs in utero may lead to club feet, and spina bifida is associated with latex sensitivity. Other symptoms include weakness, paralysis, and lack of sensation in the lower body, as well as a lack of bowel and bladder function.

Patient education emphasizing the importance of folic acid in pregnancy reduces the risk of neural tube defects. Folic acid is required for proper neural tube formation, and supplementation one month prior to conception and through the first trimester reduces the risk of defects. Blood screening and amniocentesis are used to detect spina bifida prenatally. Delivery by cesarean section prevents damage to meningocele or myelomeningocele, which reduces the risk of infection. Meningocele and myelomeningocele should be kept moist with saline gauze until the opening is surgically closed, typically within 24 hours of birth. Care should be taken to prevent stool from contacting the wound. To monitor hydrocephalus, head circumference should be measured regularly. Parents should be educated in techniques to minimize infection risks, maintain healthy skin, and improve neuromuscular function.

Each of these terms describes possible manifestations of spina bifida occulta, which occurs due to abnormal closure of the neural tube during fetal development.
- Lipomyelomeningocele - fatty benign tumors that typically form along the lumbar spine.
- Dermal sinus - openings or tracts in the back that extend through the dura to the spinal cord.
- Diastematomyelia – also known as split chord, the spinal cord is divided lengthwise.
- Tethered cord - the spinal cord forms an attachment at some point along the spinal canal, which causes stretching and stress on the cord with growth and movement.

Neonatal hydrocephalus

Hydrocephalus is an accumulation of cerebral spinal fluid due to overproduction, impaired absorption, or obstructed flow to absorption sites; cerebral ventricles are enlarged. In communicating hydrocephalus, cerebral spinal fluid circulation is maintained, but non-communicating hydrocephalus caused by blockage. Congenital causes of hydrocephalus include Dandy-Walker (cerebellar) malformation, Arnold-Chiari malformation, cerebral spinal fluid circulatory system occlusion or malformation, and Bickers-Adams syndrome. Head circumference in infants may increase by greater than 2 cm per week, and they may have apnea, bradycardia, and vomiting. Infants may receive ventriculoperitoneal shunts, and should be monitored for infection, catheter/shunt obstruction, and hemorrhage. Cooling procedures and antibiotic administration may be required if infection does develop. Parent education includes shunt care.

Alzheimer's disease

Over the first 2 to 4 years of symptomatic disease progression, patients may experience subtle forgetfulness and loss of concentration early on, but these are often overlooked or compensated for with written reminders. Progressively more difficulty with cognitive tasks and learning new skills or information, as well as declining interest in surroundings is observed. These functional deficits may affect work performance.

In mild to moderate Alzheimer's disease, which may take 2 to 12 years to develop, memory continues to decline. Patients may need assistance with remembering to pay bills, take medications, conduct personal hygiene, or do household chores. Patients lose track of possessions or get lost in well-known surroundings, including their own home. They have difficulty following instructions and begin to show language impairments. Behavior lacks inhibition and patients may be irritable, anxious or overly active. Sleep patterns are disrupted and they become more active at night. All of these problems worsen with time, progressing to needing assistance with routine decision making, such as picking out clothes, and to requiring intensive help with personal care. Incontinence develops.

The final stages of Alzheimer's disease typically occur within 8 to 10 years, but may delay as long as 25 years. Language abilities, including vocabulary, decline and disappear. Patients do not eat well and lose weight. Muscle control progressively declines, first affecting walking, then sitting, and eventually ability to hold up the head and move facial muscles. They become bedridden and completely dependent for care. Aspiration pneumonia is the primary cause of death.

Age is the primary risk factor in diagnosing Alzheimer's disease. Presentation of dementia conforming to an identified set of characteristics is typically used to identify patients with Alzheimer's. These criteria include cognitive deficits: both learning and recall are affected, as well as language, voluntary motor function, or executive function. These deficits must interfere with regular activities and other neurological causes must be ruled out. Development of the disease has hereditary components, and genetic markers, such as ApoE e4 may be useful for confirming diagnosis. MRI may reveal neural atrophy, but true diagnosis of Alzheimer's disease occurs postmortem, when the presence of amyloid plaques and neurofibrillary tangles in the brain is confirmed.

Symptoms of Alzheimer's disease may be alleviated with a class of drugs called anticholinesterases. By inhibiting acetylcholinesterase, the enzyme that breaks down the neurotransmitter acetylcholine in the synaptic cleft, these drugs promote cholinergic activity. They include tacrine, donepezil, rivastigmine, and galantamine. Side effects of these drugs include nausea and vomiting. Memantine, a drug that works by a different mechanism, was also recently approved. Memantine is a NMDA-type glutamate receptor antagonist, and combinations of memantine with other drugs may also be effective. Side effects include hallucinations, confusion, and dizziness. Other pharmacotherapy may be prescribed for depression, psychosis, or agitation. These include serotonin reuptake inhibitor antidepressants, haloperidol, and benzodiazepines.

The burden of Alzheimer's disease patient care falls primarily on family. The progressive and dehumanizing nature of the disease make care prolonged and taxing. Caregiver education, both orally and written, is important to ensure that they are aware of various resources and support groups. Information may also include strategies to prevent injury, enhance communication, or maintain appropriate social contact at each stage of the disease. Ideas to deal with sleep issues or wandering may be discussed. Caregivers should be aware of and anticipate forthcoming behavioral issues, and thus be prepared to cope with them. This includes the pending loss of decision-making abilities, and families should be encouraged to deal with financial and end-of-life issues while the patient can still participate. Sympathize with family and caregiver stress and provide options for coping.

Alzheimer's patients are primarily cared for in the home, by family. Caregiver education both improves care and eases the burden on family, postponing institutional placement of the patient. Providing support and information, particularly about what to expect and suggestions for proactive decision making, are important nursing functions. The progression of Alzheimer's requires an adaptable care plan, as physical abilities and mental capacity decline. In collaboration with the caregiver, nursing interventions may include suggestions for environmental modifications to prevent injury, or tools to cope with altered communication abilities. Assist the family with preparations to deal with likely problems such as forgetfulness and wandering. In early stages, the patient should be encouraged to continue with as many hobbies and normal activities for as long as possible. Structured activities including scheduled exercise help to regulate sleeping patterns.

Dystonia

Dystonia is a broad term for movement disorders characterized by persistent muscle contraction patterns resulting in abnormal posturing. Specific causes vary, but nervous system dysfunction in movement centers including the cerebral cortex and basal ganglia are likely to be involved. Primary dystonia is idiopathic or genetic, and secondary dystonia has an attributable cause, such as trauma or a medication side effect. Focal dystonias involve specific muscle groups, such as the neck, eyes, eyelids, and jaw. In cervical dystonia, abnormal rotation and flexion of the neck is observed. The eyelids blink uncontrollably or remain shut, effectively causing blindness, in blepharospasm. Oromandibular dystonia involves the jaw and tongue, causing deformation of the mouth. In spasmodic dystonia, the larynx is affected, often forcing a whisper. Oculogyric crisis involves the eyes, and usually the neck and jaw, causing the eyes to look up and converge, neck flexion and jaw opening or clenching. Focal dystonia may expand to include adjacent parts (segmental dystonia), or become generalized.

Dystonia treatment focuses on symptom management, and also aims to minimize disability by preserving walking function and hand use. Muscle contractions may be controlled with anticholinergic drugs, baclofen, or botulinum injections into or surgical denervation of affected muscles. Deep brain stimulation may improve symptoms of generalized dystonia. Some forms of the disease are termed "dopa-responsive," and these patients respond well to dopaminergic treatment with L-DOPA (levodopa). Although life expectancy is normal, increased disability accompanies the progression of the disease. Patients may experience depression or anxiety brought on by increasing disability or disfigurement. This may be managed pharmacologically, and encouraging social interaction can also help alleviate these feelings.

Parkinson's disease

Parkinson's disease is a movement disorder classically characterized by the presence of resting tremor, bradykinesia, and rigidity. Age is the primary risk factor, although exposure to pesticides and other environmental pollutants also appear to increase risk. It is a neurodegenerative disease, and the most prominent degeneration occurs in the substantia nigra, a dopamine-producing region of the midbrain with important regulatory functions in the production of movement. This dopamine depletion in the brain accounts for most symptoms, and indeed, the most effective alleviation of motor symptoms occurs with artificial elevation of dopamine levels. Other characteristics include a paucity of facial expression, anosmia (decreased ability to smell), drooling, sleep disturbances, and orthostatic hypotension. Loss of dopamine also contributes to cognitive decline and dementia in later stages of the disease. Neurological testing and movement assessment are primary diagnostic tools.

Pharmacotherapy for Parkinson's disease is complex and will vary through the course of treatment. Drug options include L-DOPA (levodopa), a dopamine precursor that is taken up in the brain and converted into dopamine, dopamine agonist drugs, and other drugs that support dopaminergic activity. Combinations of these drugs are frequently used. Sleepiness is a side effect of all dopaminergic drugs, and this may affect independence, especially when it comes to driving. Dopamine agonists such as pergolide, pramipexole, bromocriptine, and ropinirole lead to fewer dyskinesias than L-DOPA, but may also cause hallucinations. Selegiline supports dopaminergic function by blocking the activity of monoamine oxidase B, an enzyme that breaks down dopamine. Anticholinergics are also used to decrease involuntary muscle contractions. To optimize L-DOPA absorption into the bloodstream, it should not be taken with a meal high in protein. With time, formerly adequate doses lose their effectiveness, leading to more frequent dosing. Dopaminergic therapy also causes dyskinesias to develop, which can also be debilitating. Adjusting treatment to balance symptom control with dyskinesia production is important to effective disease management.

Common symptoms can be effectively managed. Orthostatic hypotension may be improved with increased salt intake or compression stockings. Increased fiber intake and laxatives can relieve constipation. The symptomatic combination of bradykinesia and rigidity leads to postural instability, increasing the likelihood of falling. They may also have difficulty swallowing, leading to choking. Appropriate precautions should be made to prevent injury. Anxiety is another common occurrence, and patients should be reassured that this is part of the disease. Depression and dementia may also occur, but care should be taken in their pharmacotherapy to avoid contraindications. Aspiration pneumonia is a common cause of death in the late stages of Parkinson's disease.

The progression of the disease eventually overcomes the ability of formerly effective drugs to alleviate symptoms, and severe motor side effects, termed dyskinesias, develop. Effectively managing motor symptoms while minimizing dyskinesias is the aim of Parkinson's disease therapy.

When pharmacotherapy no longer prevents either disease symptoms or dyskinesias from interfering with daily life, surgical options may be explored. These include deep brain stimulation and focal ablation of certain brain centers that malfunction without dopamine in Parkinson's disease. Electrical stimulation of the subthalamic nucleus regulates overactivity in the basal ganglia, supporting voluntary control of movement. Implantation of stimulating devices has the advantage of being adjustable, but is also susceptible to infection and malfunction. Likewise, the purpose of pallidotomy, or surgical removal of the globus pallidus internus, is to regulate the function of motor signaling pathways. This type of surgery has fewer complications, but is not adjustable.

Dyskinesia

A major side effect of Parkinson's disease pharmacotherapy is the development of dyskinesias, or repetitive uncontrolled movements. Dyskinesias, like the motor symptoms of the disease, interfere with normal function. As the brain adjusts to treatment, doses that have been effective for years no longer manage the symptoms, precipitating more frequent dosage. In addition, progressive sensitivity to dopamine therapy leads to aberrant motor system stimulation and abnormal, uncontrolled movement. For these reasons, therapy may be delayed until symptoms interfere with daily living. Once therapy is necessary, the choice of drug to start on may be influenced by patient age: younger patients are likely to be on therapy for many years and starting with dopamine agonists, rather than L-DOPA, may delay the onset of dyskinesia. Older patients may have more difficulty dealing with the hallucinations associated with dopamine agonists, and might do better starting with L-DOPA.

Geriatric thermoregulation

Thermoregulatory functions are altered in older patients. Their autonomic nervous system is less responsive to the need to adjust, and so they are less able to maintain a healthy temperature. In addition to impaired neural communication to activate adaptive systems, older patients have less physical ability to sweat and shiver. Head injury may further impair thermoregulation. Patients are considered mildly hypothermic at 32° to 35° C, moderately hypothermic at 28° to 32° C, and severely cold at less than 28° C. Hyperthermia occurs at temperatures over 40° C. Monitoring temperature and related functions is critical to overall care. Impaired thermoregulation may affect mental status and comfort, impacting diagnostic assessment or responsiveness to other treatments.

Geriatric motor deficits

Special consideration should be given to the motor capabilities of older patients. Muscle tissue is lost with age, and nerve cell function also declines. Trauma, disease, and exercise habits all contribute to neuromuscular function and their effects accumulate in the elderly. Older patients experience a loss of grip strength, followed by fatigue and more general loss of strength. Peripheral sensation may also be dulled, leading to slowed reflexes and increased burns and abrasions. These deficits increase the risk of falls, and the elderly are particularly susceptible to injury from falling. Developing an exercise plan to maintain muscle and bone mass, joint health, and coordination will prevent injury and delay disability due to neuromuscular decline.

Acute confusional state

Elderly patients that demonstrate acute behavioral changes in awareness or attention, perception, speech intelligibility, or psychomotor function may be in an acute confusional state. Otherwise known as ACS or delirium, disorientation is also common with this condition. It is differentiable from dementia due to the abrupt onset, and can occur simultaneously with other psychiatric disorders. Cardiovascular problems or other systemic conditions bring on the confusional state, not neurological problems. These conditions include metabolic imbalances brought on by dehydration or malnutrition. In addition, pain, and changes in drugs, sleep cycles, or sensory stimulation may precipitate delirium. Pharmacological management may be gradually implemented to moderate fear and delusions. A structured environment can induce calm in an agitated patient and controlled stimulation is helpful for a lethargic patient. The presence of family can be reassuring.

Geriatric depression

Depression is a mood disorder affecting many elderly patients. It has high prevalence in both the elderly and their caregivers, affecting their ability to function in daily tasks and worsening other impairments. Depression increases the risk of suicide. Chronic illnesses with associated disability are linked with development of depression. Although some symptoms may overlap, depression is separable from other mental states such as dementia, and should be independently addressed. Drug treatment in combination with psychological therapy and emotional support can effectively manage depression. Selective serotonin reuptake inhibitors are effective geriatric antidepressants, as they are better tolerated than other types. Encouraging social and physical activity can also alleviate symptoms.

Geriatric anxiety

Although mild anxiety is an informative emotional response to unfamiliar situations, severe feelings of anxiety, worry, and dread may disrupt daily activities and interfere with treatment for other problems. Acute anxiety may also signify the onset of infection or other health problems. Although anxiety is frequently observed in the elderly, it may be observed in younger populations as well. In addition to anxious feelings, symptoms include panic, seclusion, impaired concentration and organization, and restlessness. Increased heart rate, high blood pressure, increased perspiration, urinary frequency and diarrhea may also be present. Symptoms of anxiety are often increased in the evening, and are sometimes described as "sundowning." Some pharmacological treatments are helpful to calm anxious patients, but interactions with other treatments must be considered. Antidepressants may manage some symptoms. Behavioral interventions include relaxation techniques, massage, and diversional activities.

Geriatric medication considerations

Many physiological functions are altered in older adults, altering the way drugs are absorbed and metabolized in the body. Unpredictable dose effects and altered toxicity profiles also affect pharmacotherapy in the elderly. Age-related changes in renal and hepatic function, as well as altered lean tissue to fat tissue ratios affect the absorption, distribution, and excretion of drugs. Disease states also impact these parameters by altering cardiovascular, pulmonary, and gastrointestinal function. Hydration and nutritional status may be variable in the elderly, further affecting pharmacokinetics. In addition, older patients are more likely to be taking multiple medications, and interactions among these drugs must be considered. Many elderly patients take several prescribed medications daily, as well as occasional over-the-counter drugs.

Multiple disease states

Older patients are likely to sustain several chronic diseases, including hypertension, arthritis, and diabetes. These conditions are important considerations in patient care, and also affect patient independence and functionality. Adding neuromotor or other neurological problems to existing functional limitations may cause synergistic impairments. These deficits may impact job performance and social interactions, as well as general independence and activities of daily living. Altered functional abilities impact overall health, and observing these changes may indicate compromised health status. Additive disease states contribute to frailty and increase the risk of falling, injury, and illness. Hospitalization and institutionalization are also more common for these patients.

Infection

Immune system function, like many physiological functions, declines with age. Existing medical conditions may also impact the ability of the elderly patient to fight infection. Age, disease, or neurological function related impairments that affect mobility might compromise hygiene of both person and environment. Infrequent washing or inappropriate food preparation or utensil cleanliness, for example, may increase the risk of incurring infection. Typical signifiers of infection, including fever or increased white blood cell counts, may not be present in the elderly. Changes in behavioral state, such as agitation, confusion, or decreased appetite may indicate possible infection. Most cases of pneumonia occur in those over 65 years of age, and it is commonly contracted by both institutionalized patients and those staying at home. Swallowing problems, which accompany many neuroscience cases, should be carefully monitored to prevent aspiration and pneumonia. Monitoring of indwelling catheters is important to prevent bladder and urinary tract infections. Skin integrity is also compromised in the elderly, increasing susceptibility to tissue infections.

Benign essential tremor

These high frequency oscillatory movements are bilateral, and involve the hands and forearms. In contrast to Parkinsonian rest tremor, benign essential tremor occurs while a posture is maintained (postural) or while carrying out voluntary movements (kinetic). It is the most common movement disorder. Alcohol may improve symptoms, and tremor is not present during sleep. Most patients are elderly, but a peak in age of onset also occurs in the second decade of life. Genetic predisposition accounts for most cases. Progression of the disorder is generally very slow, but is disabling for some patients. Stress, fatigue, or concurrent health problems may worsen tremor, and it may interfere with occupational or living activities. A variety of medications may lessen tremor somewhat, but surgical interventions such as thalamotomy of the ventral intermediate nucleus or deep brain stimulation have greater success. Limiting caffeine and stress help to control tremor, and occupational disability may be overcome with adaptive devices.

Peripheral neuropathy

Peripheral neuropathy is a condition in which the patient experiences the chronic sensation of pain, tingling, numbness or other dysesthesias in the periphery, often in the feet or hands. Nerve damage caused by impact, chemical toxins (such as some HIV drugs), or compression precipitate this disorder, but the primary cause is thought to be demyelination. Diabetes, HIV, and peripheral nerve trauma are all predisposing factors, and increasing age also increases prevalence. In addition to uncomfortable sensations, patients will also have weakness, and normal sensation may be reduced. This combination of problems causes patients to have difficulty walking or using their hands. They are at increased risk of injury from falls, and may need a supportive brace to complete manual tasks. Pain is an ongoing concern, and is primarily managed pharmacologically. Exercise, physical therapy, and proper nutrition can slow functional decline and also help to alleviate pain.

Vertebral compression fracture

Bones weakened due to trauma, tumors, hemangioma, and especially osteoporosis, are susceptible to breakage, including the vertebrae. Back pain, decreased function, and deformity may result from vertebral compression fracture. Age and female sex increase the risk of developing osteoporosis, as do diabetes mellitus, asthma, emphysema, liver cirrhosis, chronic renal disease, rheumatoid arthritis, organ transplant, hyperthyroidism, vitamin D deficiency, premenopausal bilateral ovariectomy and premature menopause. Some medications, including steroids and anticonvulsants also increase the risk of osteoporosis and bone fracture. Measures to prevent initial and further fractures include calcium and vitamin D supplementation, and weight-bearing exercise programs to increase bone density.

Degenerative disc disease

With age, intervertebral discs dehydrate and lose blood supply. These changes in composition lead to deterioration of the disc, which increases the risk of disc herniation, and diminishes the cushioning ability of the disc, which may lead to vertebral slippage (spondylolisthesis), or spinal stenosis. Degeneration of the outer portion of disc tissue, the annulus fibrosis, allows the inner segment, the nucleus pulposus, to herniate. Only the outer third of the disc is innervated, and herniation or other stimuli cause back pain. Radiographic evidence of degeneration may not always result in symptoms, but disc degeneration typically causes back pain, limits function and contributes to disability. Severe degeneration is associated with the formation of bony outgrowths, or bone spurs, on the adjacent vertebrae. Such osteophyte formation due to disc degeneration is termed spondylosis.

Treatment for degenerative disc disease
Conservative or nonsurgical treatment for degenerative disc disease is considered the most successful intervention, consisting of oral and injectable medication to control pain and inflammation and promote muscle relaxation and physical therapy, such as activity modification, pain management modalities, and a home exercise program. Following 6 months of conservative therapy without pain relief or in cases where the activities of daily living are extremely compromised, surgical intervention is considered. Surgery involves lumbar spine fusion, aimed at ceasing the motion at a painful segment, thereby reducing pain. Lumbar fusion can improve a patient's activity levels with decreased pain and, ultimately, his or her quality of life. In an attempt to preserve the lower back anatomy, however, artificial disc replacement is used rather than fusing the disc space; this decreases the possibility of adjacent lumbar levels breaking down due to the increased stress at the fused level.

Spondylosis

As intervertebral discs degenerate, adjacent vertebrae contact each other and form bony growths, or osteophytes. Vertebral fusion may occur, limiting function, and spinal stenosis is also likely, causing nerve irritation and further pain. Long-term vertebral stress, such as that experienced by athletes or laborers, can also lead to osteophyte formation. Back or postural deformity, neck, back, or leg pain, and disability accompany spondylosis, although some patients display no symptoms. Spondylosis often occurs in the cervical region, and neck exercises are used to increase mobility. Exercise is helpful to maintain flexibility and mobility, and weight loss can decrease the stress on vertebral joints.

Spondylolisthesis

Spondylolisthesis occurs when two vertebrae become misaligned front-to-back. It most often occurs in the lumbar back between L5 and S1 or L4 and L5. Dysplastic slippage develops with spondylolysis, or inappropriate vertebral development, which often occurs with spina bifida. Isthmic spondylolisthesis also has a developmental cause, and is associated with recurring vertebral fracture and healing cycles. Hyperthyroidism, osteoporosis, and tumor cause pathological spondylolisthesis, and trauma and disc degeneration also contribute. Spondylosis may co-occur. Nerve root irritation is likely, causing pain and possibly interfering with bowel and bladder control. The spinal cord may also be compressed, causing paralysis of the lower extremities. Postural stiffening of the back leads to characteristic gait changes. Severe pain and immobility can be treated with surgical fusion of the affected vertebrae.

<u>Treatment for degenerative lumbar spondylolisthesis</u>
Treatment for degenerative lumbar spondylolisthesis includes: (1) activity modification, (2) manual manipulation, (3) epidural injections, and (4) surgery, which is rarely needed if optimal results are already achieved. Activity modification involves a short period of rest for up to 2 days, in bed or a reclining chair, with avoidance of active exercise, prolonged standing or walking, and bending backwards. This is supplemented with cold or heat application and the administration of over-the-counter (OTC) pain relievers. Exercise is introduced with the recommendation of the medical provider to include stationary biking or warm pool therapy, gradually building to a home exercise program. Aimed at decreasing pain by mobilization of painful joints, manual manipulation is provided by chiropractors, osteopaths, and physiatrists. To decrease severe pain and increase function, epidural injections may be administered. Finally, surgery to realign the affected segment can provide stability and alleviate pressure to the affected nerve.

Degenerative spine diseases

Back pain is associated with several degenerative spine diseases. Pain may occur in cervical, thoracic or lumbar (termed lumbago) regions of the back. Primary management is achieved by minimizing aggravating behavior, as well as heat, analgesics, and medication to relieve muscle spasm and inflammation. Lifestyle changes such as smoking cessation, improved nutrition and exercise habits can also control back pain. Surgical options exist for chronic sufferers, depending on the cause of the pain. Vertebral fusion and intradiscal electrothermal therapy (IDET), in which heat causes the intervertebral disc annulus to contract and destroys pain-sensing nerves, are surgical options to alleviate pain. As with other postoperative situations, surgical dressings, pain medication, and patient neurological function should be monitored. Patients may have lingering leg problems. A brace may be prescribed, and activity should be supervised.

Spinal stenosis

Spinal stenosis is narrowing of the spinal canal. Its occurrence increases with age and affects women more than men. It develops with intervertebral disc degeneration, osteoarthritis, and spondylolisthesis. This condition, usually found in the lower back, can lead to irritation and compression of the nerve roots and spinal cord, resulting in pain and weakness in the lower back and extremities, and loss of bowel and bladder control. Cervical stenosis may also restrict arterial flow in the spinal column. Activities that increase vertebral pressure, and thus pressure on the nerve roots, such as standing for long periods of time, aggravate painful symptoms. Anti-inflammatories, muscle relaxants, and rest reduce stress on the nerves and may provide temporary relief. Surgical decompression can be achieved with vertebral fusion can in the cases of spondylolisthesis, and removal of impinging bone or tissue can also restore nerve function. These treatments may not relieve back pain, but should alleviate symptoms of the legs, bowel, and bladder.

Dementia

Dementia refers to a state of declined social, cognitive, and memory abilities compared with premorbid intellectual function. It limits normal occupational and social functioning. Alzheimer's disease accounts for most dementias, followed by vascular and other degenerative causes. Many dementias are reversible, including those caused by drugs, vitamin deficiencies, and metabolic disorders. Although mild memory loss occurs with normal aging, progressive changes in cognitive function, personality, personal care habits, and ability to perform previously usual tasks characterize dementia. Cognitive changes include: forgetfulness, poor concentration, confusion, difficulty finding the right word, or understanding written language. Frequently getting lost, inattention to personal care, and difficulty with problem solving or regular home or occupational activities are also behavioral changes of note. Patients with dementia also exhibit mood swings, anxiety, fearfulness, depression and social withdrawal, as well as loss of social inhibition, sexual aggressiveness, and agitation.

Vascular dementia

Alzheimer's disease causes over half of dementias, and vascular dementia accounts for about a quarter. Vascular dementia refers to dementia arising from neural damage of cardio- or cerebrovascular origin. As with all dementias, changes in cognitive and day-to-day function are observed with vascular dementia. Multi-infarct dementia occurs with cumulative neural damage. In contrast to Alzheimer's disease dementia, multi-infarct dementia has a sharper onset and correlated progression. Imaging can reveal multiple infarcts, and other focal neurological deficits, such as hemiparesis, accompany the dementia. Vascular and Alzheimer's disease dementias may co-occur. When multiple infarcts occur mainly in the white matter, the frontal lobes may be infarcted or show decreased activity, and a different set of symptoms is observed. In diffuse white matter dementia, also termed subcortical arteriosclerotic encephalopathy or Binswanger's disease, confusion, apathy and forgetfulness are followed by behavioral changes and gait disorders. Slow progression may lead to urinary incontinence and difficulty speaking.

Vascular dementia treatment

Hypertension, coronary artery disease, and diabetes, primary risk factors for stroke, are thus also implicated in development of vascular dementia. Dementia due to damage of vascular origin is approached in the same way as stroke generally: behavioral modifications and medical management. Smoking cessation, improved diet and exercise habits, management of cholesterol levels, diabetes, and blood pressure all reduce the risk of infarct. Antiplatelet and anticoagulant medications may also be of use. Vascular dementia patients are at higher risk for falls than patients with other dementias, and care should be taken to minimize risk of injury.

Ménière's disease

Symptoms associated with Ménière's disease typically occur in the fifth decade of life. Excessive endolymph volume and pressure in the inner ear are thought to affect vestibular and cochlear function of cranial nerve VIII, leading to both balance and hearing problems. Classic symptoms include vertigo, progressive deafness, tinnitus (ringing in the ears), and a sensation of fullness in the ear. The symptoms occur periodically, with vertigo lasting minutes or hours. Patients often experience anxiety between bouts. Hearing loss may begin before attacks of vertigo, and, along, with tinnitus, gradually worsens to the point of complete deafness. Hearing loss is usually unilateral, but affects some patients bilaterally. Nystagmus, or rhythmic eye movements, is often observed, and vertigo may cause nausea and vomiting.

Patients with Ménière's disease usually receive treatment in the home setting. Vertigo may prevent the patient from standing or walking. During attacks, patients should be encouraged to stay in bed and try different positions to minimize vertigo. Fall and injury prevention are concerns. Medication to control nausea and vomiting may be helpful. Conditions such as ear or respiratory infections, head trauma, and fluid retention (including that associated with pregnancy and menstruation) may cause or exacerbate symptoms. Low-salt diet, diuretics, and antihistamines may lower pressure in the inner ear and alleviate symptoms. Sedatives may reduce anxiety between attacks. Nursing evaluation of symptom management is important to optimizing drug treatment. Patients with complete unilateral deafness and frequent incapacitating attacks may benefit from surgical labyrinthectomy, which destroys the vestibular mechanism of one ear. Sectioning the vestibular portion of cranial nerve VIII is another surgical option to eliminate vertigo.

Down syndrome

Down syndrome is a developmental disorder caused by the presence of a third copy or other abnormality with chromosome 21. A characteristic set of physical and behavioral traits define the syndrome. Physical features of people with Down syndrome include a short, broad head with flattened occipital shape, flattened bridge of the nose, large tongue, short fingers, less than average height, and immature genitalia. Many also have heart malformations. Mental development is usually mildly to moderately retarded, but many are able to learn basic vocational skills. Risk factors include mother under 16 or over 35, or pregnancy after several other pregnancies. Thyroid or pituitary deficiencies in the mother may also contribute. Prenatal amniocentesis can be used to identify Down syndrome babies.

Intervention strategies for Down syndrome
Upon determining intervention strategies to aid in phonological development, four aspects of the phonology of Down syndrome should be considered: (1) prelinguistic stage, (2) transition to speech, (3) single-word phonology, and (4) phonological characteristics of speech in conversation. Additional factors, such as hearing loss and differences in anatomy and physiology, play a role in the cognitive deficit in phonological development, making it difficult to perceive and produce speech and, ultimately, to communicate with society. As there are limited resources for special education involving speech therapy, articulation therapy is a high priority aimed at childhood through adolescence. Improvement of aspects of speech, such as segmental and suprasegmental aspects, ultimately improves the individual's intelligibility and promotes a sense of worth by being understood. Articulation therapy progresses from single words to the development of articulation skills and finally to conversational speech.

Craniosynostosis

Synostosis is defined as a union of adjacent bones. Craniosynostosis involves premature skull suture closure in the newborn. When only one suture is affected (single-suture synostosis) and the remaining sutures close normally, a normal newborn results. However, multiple synostosis involves the premature closure of multiple sutures (i.e., one to three or more sutures). If no other problems exist, this is called nonsyndromic, multisuture synostosis; however, syndromes, such as Crouzon,

Apert, and Pfeiffer, are accompanied by systemic problems, in addition to multiple synostosis. Four types of synostosis may develop, depending on the affected suture: (1) sagittal, involving the midline sagittal suture; (2) coronal, involving the coronal suture of the lateral head from the anterior fontanelle to above the ear; (3) metopic, involving the midline suture from the anterior fontanelle to the root of the nose; and (4) lambdoidal, involving a flattening of the back of the skull.

Treatment for craniosynostosis
With a diagnosis of craniosynostosis, frequent provider follow-up visits for head measurements are warranted to monitor for growth failure and related clinical manifestations from the effects of increased intracranial pressure. Surgical treatment is the only treatment choice with two surgical procedures available: (1) to relieve the cranial sutures that are fused and (2) to create a suture line with an incision of the skull bone. The first procedure involves an open incision on the skull bone surface, after which the skull bones are repositioned to correct any asymmetry. Hardware, which is absorbed over time, may be necessary to secure the repositioned skull bones in place. The second procedure involves the insertion of an endoscopic device through a small incision, releasing the fused suture to allow more flexibility. In addition to surgical correction of the craniosynostosis, further primary and secondary surgeries may be indicated to improve any resultant facial abnormalities.

Friedreich's ataxia

Friedreich's ataxia (spinocerebellar degeneration) is a rare disease that attacks muscles and the heart. It is caused by changes or a defect in the gene, frataxin (FXN), located on chromosome 9, which causes excessive production of the DNA, the GAA trinucleotide repeat, and which is directly related to a young age of onset and speed of progression. Brain and spinal cord structures control muscle movement, coordination, and some sensory functions. Symptoms of Friedreich's ataxia are the result of wear on these structures and typically begin in childhood before puberty, including the following: vision changes, especially with color; jerky eye movements; loss of hearing; speech impairment; spinal changes, such as scoliosis or kyphoscoliosis; uncoordinated movement or ataxia, which worsens with time; unsteady gait; muscle weakness; loss of balance and coordination with resultant falls; decreased sensation of vibrations and no reflexes in the lower limbs; and foot problems, including high arches and hammertoes.

Treatment for Friedreich's ataxia
As there is no known cure or effective treatment for Friedreich's ataxia, medical management is aimed at the maintenance of optimal functioning by treating the complications of diabetes, heart disease, and heart failure and the inability to maintain mobility. These interventions include: (1) treatment of diabetes and heart disease with medication; (2) physical therapy to prolong the use of the patient's arms and legs; (3) orthotics (e.g., braces, surgery for orthopedic problems, such as foot deformities and scoliosis); (4) durable medical equipment, such as wheelchairs, typically within 15 years of the onset of the disease, or walking aids; (5) speech therapy; and (6) counseling. As the disease progresses, the patient will experience increasing difficulty performing the activities of daily living. The Friedreich's Ataxia Research Alliance keeps a worldwide registry of patients afflicted with Friedreich's ataxia and funds ongoing research that attempts to understand this disease and to discover any new treatments.

ADHD

Attention Deficit Hyperactivity Disorcer (ADHD) is a disorder most commonly reported in childhood. It is typified by inattention, hyperactivity, and impulsiveness. People with ADHD have difficulty focusing on tasks or stimuli appropriately and are often distracted. They may also display learning disabilities, obsessive-compulsive behavior, antisocial behavior, depression, and are prone to substance abuse. The cause of ADHD is unclear, but the executive functions of the frontal lobes appear to be impaired, and the neurotransmitter dopamine has been implicated. Observing behavior in different settings for characteristic distractibility, difficulty following instructions, and restlessness are critical for diagnosis. Fetal alcohol syndrome and some medications, such as anticonvulsants and antihypertensives, can also cause symptoms of inattention, hyperactivity, and impulsiveness.

ADHD is often treated with behavioral or a combination of behavioral and drug therapies. The goal of therapy is to optimize functionality. Proactive measures to limit distractions, organize time, and self-monitoring techniques to respond to different situations are helpful for adults, and children can also benefit from quiet, structured environments. Lists can help with staying on task. Medications that stimulate the monoamine systems of dopamine and norepinephrine are effective in reducing hyperactivity and improve attention. These drugs may also affect sleep patterns, appetite, and cause stomach or headaches. Regular monitoring at home and school, rather than just periodic clinical assessments, is important to evaluate and adjust coping strategies appropriately.

Chronic pain

Unlike acute pain, which signals immediate tissue damage or potentially damaging stimuli, chronic pain has no biological function. It persists beyond the presentation of noxious stimuli and time course of healing, generally considered 4-6 weeks after acute injury. Chronic pain may occur continuously or recur, spanning months or years. It is associated with depression and long-term disability. Describing and evaluating the pain is necessary to judge therapeutic efficacy. Pain history, including descriptions of onset, location, intensity, and level of interference with normal activities should be collected. History of treatment, including methods and degree of relief achieved, should also be included. Characteristics of the pain, such as quality (sharp, dull), variation with time or activity, periodicity, and aggravating factors should also be noted. Pain rating scales are useful in gauging the pain experience of an individual.

The participation of the patient and caregivers is essential for optimal pain management, and cooperative development of a pain control plan along with the health care provider is a first step. A combination of both pharmacological and behavioral therapies is critical, and monitoring the effectiveness of control measures is necessary to appropriately adjust the care plan. Physical therapies to alleviate pain include hot or cold application, which affect blood flow and muscle tone. Exercise is important to regulate muscle tension and maintain function. Transcutaneous electrical nerve stimulation (TENS) is thought to modulate nociceptive transmission. Relaxation, meditation, and distraction are effective behavioral strategies. Analgesic medications may be opioid or non-narcotic; non-narcotic drugs are typically used for chronic pain to avoid issues of tolerance and abuse. Antidepressants complement other analgesics by diminishing the pain experience, and anticonvulsants reduce nociceptive transmission. Counseling and peer support groups can aid in coping.

Neurogenic pain

Neurogenic pain, or pain of neural origin, is chronic pain caused by nerve damage. Several spinal disorders, including spinal cord tumors, intervertebral disc degeneration, spinal stenosis, and trauma lead to spinal cord or nerve root irritation or compression, as do entrapment syndromes such as carpal tunnel. Traumatic nerve injury may result in causalgia (also called Complex Regional Pain syndrome-II, CRPS-II), a syndrome including hyperpathia and psychomotor dysfunction. Phantom pain, or pain perceived to originate from a body part that no longer exists (as after amputation), is inherently neurogenic. Neurogenic chronic pain may be managed surgically. Rhizotomy destroys the dorsal sensory nerve root, thereby removing all related sensation, while sparing the ventral motor fibers. Cordotomy produces extensive unilateral analgesia by lesioning the spinothalamic tract. Pre- and postoperative assessments include describing and rating pain, and acute postoperative pain must be controlled. Patients should be educated about appropriate expectations for pain relief.

End-of-life care

Neuroscience conditions affect people across the lifespan, and nurses may be involved in end-of-life care decisions. Ethical use of life-sustaining interventions, such as ventilators and feeding tubes, is continually in question. Competent patients may decide to discontinue ventilator support. Similarly, competent patients or designees may opt to discontinue artificial hydration and nutrition, or that provided by means other than the mouth (assisted oral intake is not considered artificial) if anticipated burdens outweigh the possibility of sustained quality of life. When prolongation of life is not possible, optimizing comfort and minimizing pain are the focus. Nursing assessment of pain is important to assure its adequate control. Brain death, or complete loss of neural function, is diagnosed clinically with reference to unresponsiveness, lack of brain-stem reflexes, and apnea. After brain death is declared, and if the patient consented, organs may be harvested for donation. Providing information, respect and support of patient and family decisions is important.

Important Terms

Spina bifida – also known as spinal dysraphism, failure of the neural tube to fuse properly during development that leads to abnormal formation of the spinal column.
Meningocele – type of spina bifida aperta in which a sac composed of dura and arachnoid protrudes through the spinal column defect, meningocele is also the name for the sac itself.
Myelomeningocele – type of spina bifida aperta in which the spinal meninges protrude beyond the spinal column and the spinal cord is also involved, myelomeningocele is also the name for the sac itself.
Degenerative disc disease – age-associated degeneration of spinal discs; increases susceptibility to disc tissue herniation, spondylolisthesis, and spinal stenosis; causes neck or back pain.
Spondylolisthesis – slippage of vertebrae relative to each other; disc degeneration is a predisposing factor; may impinge on spinal cord space and cause nerve irritation.

Spondylosis – formation of bone spurs on vertebrae due to disc degeneration; may lead to vertebral fusion and spinal stenosis.

Spinal stenosis – narrowing of the spinal column space that accommodates the spinal cord; may occur with spondylolisthesis or spondylosis; increases likelihood of nerve compression.

Vertebral compression fracture – spinal vertebra breakage usually attributable to bone fragility; causes back pain and has several age-linked risk factors.

Ménière's disease – balance disorder characterized by recurrent bouts of vertigo, progressive hearing loss, and tinnitus.

Benign paroxysmal positional vertigo – brief episodes of vertigo that occur during changes of the position of the head as with turning over or looking up; due to inappropriate otolith signaling relative to actual head position.

Labyrinthitis – infection of the inner ear, can cause imbalance.

Vestibular neuronitis - infection of vestibular nerves, can cause imbalance.

Vertigo – sensation of spinning, major symptom of balance disorders.

Dizziness – broad term describing light-headed sensation of unsteadiness or imbalance, may include vertigo.

Nociceptor – nerve associated with detection of noxious stimuli and triggering the sensation of pain.

Neuralgia – pain associated with damage or irritation of a nerve, usually felt in the distribution of the affected nerve.

Paresthesia - any abnormal skin sensation.

Dysesthesia – an uncomfortable or painful skin sensation, such as tingling, burning, or numbness.

Hyperesthesia – abnormally increased sensitivity to sensory stimulation (all modalities).

Hypoesthesia – abnormally diminished sensitivity to sensory stimulation.

Hyperpathia – exaggerated, painful perception of sensory stimuli.

Other Disorders

Chemical dependency

A genetic predisposition to an active addiction or a chronic, compulsive need for alcohol or drugs is thought to be linked to chemical dependency. Genetically predisposed individuals may lack adequate amounts of two brain chemicals, dopamine and serotonin. When exposed to alcohol or drugs, these individuals may experience a normal feeling not experienced before as a result of an external replacement of the depleted or lower-than-normal brain chemicals. In addition, environmental factors, such as accessibility and availability of a chemical and psychological factors, play a major role in ultimate chemical dependency. Individuals are often addicted not only to the drug itself but also to the feelings that the drug produces. Chemical dependency is progressive with worsening symptoms if untreated; it is also chronic and relapsing without a cure, ceasing only with lifestyle changes and maintenance. Chemical dependency can be fatal, as a result of the long-term impact on body organs and systems or as a result of accidental overdoses and suicides.

Treatment for chemical dependency

Treatment for chemical dependency includes inpatient/residential treatment, extended treatment, outpatient treatment, and continuing care/aftercare. With inpatient/residential treatment of at least 28 days, the patient is provided with medical management for detoxification. The outside distractions, as well as alcohol or drugs, are removed from the patient's access, allowing the patient to follow the recommended steps toward recovery. Following residential care, a patient may be transitioned to a structured, extended treatment for 2 months to 2 years duration, living in a halfway house setting, often finding employment before dismissal. With outpatient treatment, short-term intervention is provided with obviously less disruption to the patient's daily life, as the patient remains at home and may even continue to work. Finally, continuing care or aftercare is felt to be a much needed extension of the first three options, ranging from 6 months to 1 year and including group and individual counseling sessions.

Immobility interventions

Many neuroscience patients will experience immobility. Older patients may be less mobile; some patients will be unable to move due directly to neural impairment, others may be temporarily restricted after surgery. Patients are susceptible to decreased muscle strength and tone, and reduced range of motion. Skin breakdown, pressure ulcers, constipation, pneumonia, and deep venous thrombosis are all hazards associated with immobility. Proper bodily alignment, limb support, and skin care are essential preventative measures. Encouraging and supporting exercise as medically appropriate, whether passive or active, increases independence and facilitates rehabilitation. Patients requiring assistance should be turned frequently. Elastic stockings and compression air boots increase circulation, thereby preventing venous thrombosis. Elevating the lower legs with a pillow can also prevent pressure ulcer development on the heels. A bowel program may minimize constipation. Antispasmodics, botulinum, or baclofen may be prescribed to control muscle spasticity.

Gastrointestinal complications

Loss of body mass, fatigue or nausea may be indicative of gastrointestinal complications, which may arise during the care of many patients with neuroscience disorders. Such problems may hinder healing or add further medical conditions such as gastrointestinal hemorrhage. Laboratory nutritional status, in combination with physical assessments, guides interventions. Bowel sounds and abdominal tenderness, as well as swallowing ability should be assessed. Ineffective swallowing leads to aspiration. If oral intake is prohibitive, enteral or parenteral nutrition may be necessary; catheter and skin care are important supportive measures. Small, frequent meals and antacids can help prevent irritation. Monitoring intake, output, and body weight tracks the effectiveness of interventions.

Acute pain

Acute pain is generally related to tissue damage, and serves as an indicator of such injury. Severe pain may accompany such neuroscience afflictions as meningeal inflammation, stroke, subarachnoid hemorrhage, or increased intracranial pressure. Related pains may include headache, neck pain or nuchal rigidity, and back pain. Behavioral indications of pain include withdrawal, irritability, restlessness, crying or facial contortions, and protective behaviors. Monitoring these behaviors, as well as physiological signs, is indicative of pain severity and degree of relief. Location of pain should be noted, and pain rating scales used to describe the quality and severity of pain. These assessments are useful to monitor the effectiveness of interventions. Measures to ease pain include analgesic medications. Quiet, low light conditions with few disturbances promote comfort and relaxation. Repositioning or elevating the head of the bed can also alleviate pain.

Trigeminal neuralgia

Trigeminal neuralgia is usually caused by compression of the trigeminal nerve due to a neighboring atherosclerotic artery. Trauma or local infection may also contribute. This cranial nerve irritation causes intense, piercing, burning pain in the sensory distribution of the nerve. Pain occurs periodically for a few seconds over weeks, and then decreases. Motor and other sensory functions are not affected. Aneurysm, tumor, arachnoiditis, or multiple sclerosis can cause similar symptoms, but these primary causes should be ruled out. The three branches of the trigeminal nerve include the ophthalmic, maxillary, and mandibular divisions. The ophthalmic branch, which is affected less often, innervates the forehead, eyes, nose, and temples. Maxillary innervation includes the upper jaw, teeth, lip, and cheeks. Mandibular zones include the lower jaw, teeth, lip, and tongue. Patients typically have trigger zones on the face, such as an area of the cheek, forehead, lip, or gum that elicits a bout of pain when stimulated. Facial contortions, or tics, are common responses to the pain.

Drug therapy can curb pain attacks. Carbamazepine is commonly prescribed, but patients should also then be monitored for liver toxicity. Blocking individual branches of the trigeminal nerve with injections of alcohol can provide pain relief for 8 to 16 months. Percutaneous trigeminal rhizotomy is a common surgical treatment that usually effects long term pain relief. This procedure does not cause facial paralysis, is tolerated by most patients, and is associated with a very short hospital stay.

The sensory fibers that generate the pain signal are more sensitive to heat than other branches, and so thermocoagulation of these fibers relieves pain without detriment to motor function.

Trigeminal neuralgia pain and fear of pain greatly affect the behavior of patients. Facial trigger zones are sensitive to mild touch, cold, and pressure stimuli and so activities such as washing the face, brushing the teeth, talking, or chewing can elicit bouts of pain. This may prevent patients from talking, eating, or maintaining personal hygiene. Identifying trigger areas and ways to avoid stimulating them can help to prevent pain and anxiety. Patients may have nutritional and self care deficits to address, and may experience social isolation. Pain control with analgesics, sedatives, or antiepileptics may be useful. The frequency of bouts can be used to monitor the effectiveness of drug therapy. The neurological function of postoperative patients should be evaluated, including the symmetry of facial movement, extraocular movement, corneal reflex, and sense of taste. Jaw and temporal muscle function and tone should be assessed. Because surgery destroys sensory fibers, the affected side is at increased risk for injury. Caution against rubbing the eye and advise regular dental visits.

Dysomnias and parasomnias

Sleep disorders last a month or more and interfere with social or occupational functioning. Dysomnias are sleep disorders that affect the amount, restfulness, or pattern of sleep, including insomnia or hypersomnia. Many factors can cause dysomnias, some examples are: insufficient sleep, drugs, noise, depression, and time changes. Sleep deprivation can cause daytime sleepiness and affect psychological functioning. Stimulant drugs, caffeine, alcohol, antihistamines, as well as other medications, affect sleep patterns. Stress or depression can lead to sleeplessness. Shift work and jet lag contribute to circadian rhythm disorders. Dysomnias typically have onset in adulthood. Hospitalized patients may have difficulty sleeping, which may affect neurological functioning. Parasomnias also affect daily functioning and may cause emotional distress. Parasomnias include sleep disorders such as sleepwalking, sleep talking, tooth grinding, nightmares, sleep terrors, sleep paralysis, and bedwetting. These sleep behaviors may be associated with particular stages of sleep or transitions between sleep stages and waking. They affect children more often than adults.

Stages of sleep

The five stages of sleep are each associated with characteristic EEG and muscle activity patterns. They encompass the transition from waking to sleep, light and deep sleep and the dreaming state. The body cycles through each stage throughout a normal sleeping period, with the length of time spent in deep sleep stages longer earlier in the night and dream sleep stages longer later on. The first four sleep stages have no eye movement (NREM), but the fifth stage is noted for rapid eye movements (REM).

- Stage 1 occurs as someone is falling asleep.
- Stage 2 is a stage of light sleep characterized by EEG sleep spindles and K complexes. Stage 2 occurs periodically throughout the night between deep sleep and dreaming stages, and about half of sleep time is spent in stage 2.

- Stages 3 and 4 are slow wave, deep sleep stages accounting for about one-fourth of sleep time.
- In REM sleep, EEG activity increases and muscles relax except for eye movement.

Treatment for sleep apnea

Treatment for sleep apnea, if mild, includes lifestyle changes, such as smoking cessation and weight loss, and the use of an oral appliance designed to bring the jaw forward, thereby opening the throat. Treatment recommended for moderate-to-severe sleep apnea includes therapies and surgeries. Therapy modalities include the use of the following equipment: (1) continuous positive airway pressure, delivering air pressure through a mask; (2) bi-level positive airway pressure, delivering increased pressure with inhalation rather than exhalation; and (3) adaptive servo-ventilation, using pressure to normalize breathing during sleep. Surgery is indicated for the removal of excess nasal or throat tissue blocking the upper airway. Surgical options include: (1) uvulopalatopharyngoplasty (i.e., removal of the tonsils, adenoids, and posterior tissue of the mouth and the throat); (2) maxillomandibular advancement, enlarging the airway by moving the jaw forward; and (3) tracheostomy for severe, life-threatening sleep apnea.

Sleep disorders in children

Many children experience parasomnias such as sleepwalking and night terrors, and they may also have sleep apnea or narcolepsy. About a third of children, especially younger children, are thought to have nightmares, and about the same percentage demonstrate sleepwalking. Sleepwalking is most common in children under age 10. Children usually outgrow these disorders. Children also experience insomnia caused by some of the same factors that affect adults, such as anxiety or drugs. Limiting caffeine, fluids (to prevent needing to get up at night to use the bathroom), and television in the hours before bedtime can help children fall asleep, stay asleep, and lessen nightmares. Having a regular pattern at bedtime can help children to relax and prepare for bed.

Instituting good sleep hygiene, or habits, can facilitate restful sleep. These habits include waiting until feeling sleepy before going to bed, not using the bedroom for working or watching television, avoiding caffeine and limiting late evening fluid intake, getting up at the same time every morning, and exercising early in the day. Treatment of some primary disorders, such as depression or pain, may help with sleep. To facilitate sleep for hospitalized patients, decrease nighttime stimuli and schedule care to provide uninterrupted sleep periods. A sleep log for one or two weeks documenting the length of time in bed, quality of sleep, medications, and observations of family members concerning sleepwalking, movements, or snoring, can be a tool to identify behavioral patterns and involved disorders. Sleeping aids have potential of addiction and overdose, and may interact with other prescriptions. Sedatives are usually only prescribed for insomnia from temporary stress. Benzodiazepines can prevent sleep terrors and sleepwalking in children by suppressing sleep stages 3 and 4.

Toxic encephalopathies

Encephalopathies occur when systemic disease impairs brain health and function. Hepatitis or cirrhosis that compromise liver function may lead to hepatic encephalopathy. Diabetes, renal artery stenosis and various kidney diseases contribute to renal failure and uremic encephalopathy.

Hypoxic encephalopathy occurs with cardiac arrest, drowning, birth asphyxia, low blood pressure, and respiratory failure. Low serum sodium or infections may also cause encephalopathy. Symptoms of encephalopathy include incoordination, altered judgment, inattention, signs of increased intracranial pressure such as altered consciousness and coma, as well as ischemia and herniation. Encephalopathy is a manifestation of primary disease, and treatments target the root illness. Hypoxia is an emergency, and measures to restore oxygenation and respiration must occur immediately.

<u>Treatment for toxic encephalopathy</u>
Toxic encephalopathy, also known as toxic metabolic encephalopathy or metabolic encephalopathy, involves abnormal levels of water, electrolytes, liver and kidney waste products, blood sugar, sodium, vitamins, and chemicals, in addition to thyroid problems, all of which result in abnormal brain function. Abnormal brain function may be stable or static and reversible or progressive with an increased loss of brain activity. Toxic encephalopathy can also be the result of drug ingestions, medication side effects, and carbon monoxide or cyanide poisoning that affect the brain chemical neurotransmitters, decreasing overall brain function. Carbon monoxide or cyanide poisoning can hinder the transportation of oxygen by hemoglobin, leading to tissue anoxia. Treatment is dependent on the underlying cause, such as dialysis, and a kidney transplant may be required in cases of uremic poisoning. However, emergent evaluation is crucial to diagnose toxic encephalopathy accurately; to plan the treatment in order to prevent, limit, or reverse any symptoms; and to promote an optimal prognosis.

Important Terms

Cataplexy – sudden loss of muscle tone and stability; may cause total collapse for a few seconds to 30 minutes; often triggered by strong emotional responses; awareness and hearing remain functional.

Restless legs syndrome – condition in which uncomfortable paresthesias in the legs drive a compulsion to move them for relief; symptoms worsen with inactivity and at night and may disturb sleep.

Shift work disorder – circadian rhythm sleep disorder affecting people who frequently alter their sleep-wake pattern.

Sleep apnea – condition in which breathing is interrupted during sleep; may occur due to neurological problem with diaphragm control or upper airway obstruction; obstructive sleep apnea is common in the obese and typically alternates with loud snoring.

Practice Test

Practice Questions

1. Which is the most accurate statement concerning antibiotic therapy for bacterial meningitis?
   a. Treatment should not commence until the causative organism has been identified
   b. Bactericidal and bacteristatic antibiotics are equally acceptable
   c. Initial drug selection is based on the most likely organisms and should be reassessed within hours as CSF laboratory results return
   d. Antibiotic therapy should be initiated before administering any dexamethasone

2. Which of the following is NOT an important nursing intervention in the care of a patient with viral meningitis?
   a. Serial neurologic examinations to detect focal abnormalities or altered consciousness
   b. Taking steps to prevent increased intracranial pressure, such as maintaining the neck in neutral position and instituting a good bowel program to prevent the need for Valsalva
   c. Avoiding hyperthermia by keeping the room cool, applying moist cloths to the head, and administering antipyretic drugs as necessary
   d. Maintaining isolation until the patient has been afebrile without antipyretic drugs for at least 24 hours

3. The MOST important part of nursing preparation for a patient about to undergo diagnostic lumbar puncture is to:
   a. Check platelet count and coagulation studies
   b. Have the patient empty his bladder and move his bowel if possible
   c. Maintain the patient NPO for six hours or more
   d. Educate the patient about the purpose, method, and possible complications of the procedure

4. Which is the MOST important element of patient education for the patient being discharged from hospital after diagnosis and early treatment of Lyme disease?
   a. Emphasize the necessity to complete the entire course of oral antibiotics
   b. Reassure the patient that his experience with Lyme disease has conferred immunity to B. burgdorferi
   c. Instruct the patient to maintain isolation until he has completed the entire course of antibiotic therapy
   d. Alert the patient to possible long-term joint damage from the disease

5. A patient with relapsing-remitting multiple sclerosis wishes to discontinue therapy with interferon beta-1b, because she has not noticed any neurologic improvement since starting the medication two years ago. The MOST appropriate nursing response is to:
    a. Evaluate her for depression, since depression is a known side effect of interferons, as well as a likely symptom of her multiple sclerosis
    b. Help her to manage flu-like side effects by pretreating with acetaminophen or a nonsteroidal anti-inflammatory agent prior to injections
    c. Remind her that the goals of therapy are to reduce the frequency and severity of exacerbations and delay the development of disability. Provide regular phone follow-up to support her in continuing treatment
    d. Propose changing to interferon beta-1a or glatiramer acetate

6. A college student is brought to the emergency room by a dormitory roommate because of severe headache, fever, and strange behavior over the last couple of hours. There are petechiae on the skin and conjunctivae. While the patient is being prepared for lumbar puncture, what supportive measure is MOST urgent?
    a. Preparing for endotracheal intubation
    b. Providing adequate intravenous access
    c. Administering an antipyretic
    d. Educating the patient and roommate about vaccination for meningitis

7. The MOST effective way for a patient with multiple sclerosis to cool core body temperature during exercise is to:
    a. Take antipyretics, such as acetaminophen, prior to exercising
    b. Drink cool liquids
    c. Wear a cooling vest
    d. Dress lightly

8. The MOST important element of assessment of the patient hospitalized for care of worsening myasthenia is:
    a. Comprehensive assessment of respiratory function
    b. Evaluation of voice quality and volume
    c. Evaluation of extraocular muscle function
    d. Avoidance of neuromuscular-blocking drugs

9. The best dietary advice for patients with myasthenia is to:
    a. Follow a liquid diet on days when the muscles of mastication feel weak
    b. Take anticholinergic medication well in advance of every meal
    c. Never eat when fatigued
    d. Eat a mechanical soft diet and take small meals

10. Pro-active decision making about life supports such as gastrostomy for feeding or tracheostomy for ventilation is essential for patients with amyotrophic lateral sclerosis (ALS) because:
    a. Death in ALS most commonly occurs because of aspiration or respiratory failure
    b. When terminal, an ALS patient may be unable to communicate
    c. ALS is a progressive disease, and 50% of the patients die within 3 years of diagnosis
    d. For ALS patients, feeding tubes and artificial ventilation are not temporary life-saving measures that can be instituted and then withdrawn when a crisis resolves

11. The MOST essential element of respiratory monitoring of a patient hospitalized for management of Guillain-Barré syndrome is:
    a. Measuring respiratory rate at frequent intervals
    b. Checking frequently for signs of hypoxia, such as dyspnea, cyanosis, or confusion
    c. Measuring oxygenation by continuous pulse oximetry
    d. Measuring vital capacity at frequent intervals, and knowing the value at which intubation will be performed electively

12. Prevention of deep vein thrombosis in the patient hospitalized for management of Guillain-Barré syndrome is best accomplished by:

    a. Placing compression boots on the lower extremities
    b. Oral warfarin
    c. Minidoses of heparin
    d. Aspirin

13. A patient is sufficiently recovered from the acute phase of Guillain-Barré syndrome to have been successfully extubated, and now he is ready for outpatient rehabilitation. His pain, however, is intense and unrelenting, and he has concerns about his prescription for a sustained-release opioid medication. The best approach to educating this patient about his pain medication is to:
    a. Explain that a sustained-release preparation taken time-contingently, rather than pain-contingently, actually allows him to minimize his total dose of opioid and reduce side effects associated with high serum levels
    b. Warn him about the risks of respiratory suppression, since he has recently been ventilator-dependent and is still not fully recovered from Guillain-Barré syndrome
    c. Explain to the patient and family that this medication carries a risk of addiction and make sure they know the signs of addiction and the importance of communicating their concerns to the prescribing physician
    d. Encourage the patient to explore non-opioid drug options with the physician

14. The MOST suitable nursing intervention to protect the eye of a patient with Bell's palsy is to:
    a. Apply a patch
    b. Provide artificial tears for daytime instillation and protective ophthalmic ointment during sleep
    c. Teach the patient facial exercises to promote return of strength to the orbicularis oculi
    d. Recommend electrical stimulation of the involved nerve

MOMETRIX TEST PREPARATION
The World's Most Comprehensive Test Preparation Company

Dear Friend,

Thank you for ordering Mometrix products!

We take very seriously that you are entrusting your test preparation needs to us and we have meticulously prepared these materials to ensure we are offering you the most concise, relevant study aid possible. There are many resources available for your exam and we sincerely appreciate you choosing ours to help you attain the highest score within your ability to achieve. With this purchase, you are helping to provide for the many families that make up our company and in turn we hope to help you attain the results you need in order to achieve your dreams.

You are about to experience an incredible transformation. Over the next few hours, days, weeks or months of studying, you will transition from your current level of preparedness to an understanding of the exam content that you never thought possible. You hold in your hands the information you most need to know in order to succeed on your exam. Regardless of whether this is your first time to take the exam or your fifth time, our goal is to give you exactly what you need to maximize your score so you can go where you most want to go and be what you most want to be.

In addition to the products you have ordered from us, we have included a few bonuses that will help in your preparation. Be on the lookout for a special bonus website included in each product that offers additional tips and insights. In response to the test anxiety many people experience, I have also developed a free report to help you overcome this obstacle that you can access by visiting: www.mometrix.com/testanxiety.

From my family to yours, I sincerely thank you and wish you the best on your exam and every journey life has in store for you.

If you have any questions or suggestions as to how we can improve our products or service, please contact us at 800-673-8175 or support@mometrix.com.

Sincerely,

Jay Willis
Vice President of Sales
Mometrix Media LLC

P.S. – We would greatly appreciate you recommending our products to your friends and colleagues!

15. Which is the MOST FUNDAMENTAL part of patient education regarding bladder care for the patient newly diagnosed with multiple sclerosis?
   a. Instructing the patient in self-catheterization
   b. Recommending that the patient empty the bladder at regular, frequent intervals, regardless of subjective fullness
   c. Setting up a schedule for regular urine cultures
   d. Making a referral to a urologist

16. The MOST important role for nurses in PREVENTION of neurocysticercosis is:
   a. Educating patients, their families, and their other contacts about the importance of hand washing, proper handling and cooking of pork, and dietary precautions to take while traveling in endemic areas
   b. Encouraging parents to have their children properly immunized against Taenia solium
   c. Identifying asymptomatic patients for treatment by offering immunoserologic assays for T. solium antibodies
   d. Identifying all close contacts of known patients for prophylactic treatment with antihelminthic drugs

17. Nursing interventions in the care of patients with Creutzfeldt-Jakob disease include all of the following EXCEPT:
   a. Isolation precautions
   b. Psychiatric interventions
   c. Palliative care, including total care at the end of life
   d. Support for patient and family in proactively addressing end-of-life concerns

18. Once a patient has become HIV-positive, the MOST effective way to prevent AIDS-dementia complex (ADC) is which of the following?
   a. Isolation precautions to prevent opportunistic CNS infections, such as tuberculosis
   b. Prophylaxis with cholinergic medications such as donepezil
   c. Aggressive cognitive stimulation
   d. Early and sustained HAART (highly active antiretroviral therapy)

19. The MOST essential element in managing primary fatigue in multiple sclerosis is:
   a. Stimulant medication
   b. Activity pacing
   c. Occupational therapy
   d. Treatment of any underlying sleep disorder

20. The optimal position for the meningitis patient is:
   a. Neck extended
   b. Neck flexed
   c. Neck and head in neutral position
   d. Fetal position

21. For a patient anticoagulated with intravenous heparin, the MOST important laboratory parameter to follow IN ADDITION TO the PTT (partial thromboplastin time) is:
   a. The PT (prothrombin time)
   b. The platelet count
   c. The hematocrit
   d. Serum electrolytes

22. The MOST important nursing intervention to prevent rebleeding in the patient with subarachnoid hemorrhage (SAH) due to cerebral aneurysm is:
   a. Instituting a bowel program promptly upon admission
   b. Maintaining seizure precautions
   c. Placing sequential compression boots or TED hose on the lower extremities
   d. Limiting fluid intake

23. The goal of blood pressure management in the patient with an aneurysmal subarachnoid hemorrhage (SAH) awaiting definitive treatment is:
   a. Keeping blood pressure as low as possible to prevent rebleeding
   b. Keeping blood pressure as low as possible to prevent increased intracranial pressure
   c. Keeping blood pressure high enough to avoid vasodilatation and low enough to avoid cerebral edema
   d. Keeping blood pressure high enough to prevent vasospasm and low enough to avoid repeat aneurismal bleeding

24. The best response to hyponatremia in the aftermath of an intracranial aneurysmal bleed is usually:
   a. Fluid restriction and sodium restriction
   b. Fluid restriction and sodium replacement
   c. Fluid replacement and sodium replacement
   d. Sodium replacement alone

25. The most accurate statement concerning patient age and treatment outcomes for cerebral aneurysm is:
   a. For all accepted types of treatment, outcomes are not correlated with age.
   b. Above age 65, there is a higher incidence of negative treatment outcomes, even though the surgical complication rate is the same.
   c. Above age 65, the incidence of negative treatment outcomes and the incidence of surgical complications are both higher.
   d. Only ultra-soft coils have an acceptable success rate in patients over age 65.

26. Which of the following IS among the eligibility criteria for treatment of acute stroke with thrombolytic therapy?
   a. Age must be under 65
   b. The patient must also be receiving intravenous heparin
   c. Blood glucose must be under 150
   d. Symptoms must be of no more than 3 hours duration prior to starting treatment

27. In the first 24 hours following carotid endarterectomy, the MOST important vital sign to monitor and stabilize is:
    a. Temperature
    b. Heart rate and rhythm
    c. Blood pressure
    d. Respiratory rate and pulse oximetry

28. In response to a patient's loss of self-control and social inhibitions following stroke, the MOST essential nursing intervention is to:
    a. Discuss with the patient and family the likely need for psychiatric care, including pharmacotherapy
    b. Simply accept the new range of behavior and avoid judgment
    c. Explain to the patient and family that these behaviors are involuntary, resulting from brain injury
    d. Ignore the behavior

29. What is the best nutritional advice to give a patient discharged on warfarin to prevent recurrence of embolic stroke?
    a. Take a vitamin K supplement, because warfarin inhibits vitamin K
    b. Eat leafy green vegetables regularly and in moderation
    c. Do not drink more than 2 glasses of wine or 1 mixed drink per week
    d. Take an iron supplement to counteract anemia associated with silent microscopic GI bleeding

30. EARLY definitive laboratory diagnosis of herpes simplex encephalitis is possible with:
    a. CT scan of the brain
    b. A 4-fold rise in serum antibody titer
    c. Viral DNA in the cerebrospinal fluid (CSF)
    d. Characteristic temporal sharp waves on electroencephalogram (EEG)

31. While carefully monitoring the neurologic examination in a patient receiving a continuous intravenous heparin for cerebral venous thrombosis (CVT), the nurse notes an acute neurologic deficit. The immediate response should be:
    a. Discontinue the heparin and notify the physician at once
    b. Elevate the head of the bed and make sure the head remains positioned at 30 degrees
    c. Assess the patient with PTT and CT scan of the brain
    d. Obtain PTT and empirically increase the heparin infusion slightly pending the result

32. Admission to the intensive care unit is standard care for which diagnostic group, independent of neurologic status?
    a. Acute ischemic stroke
    b. Transient ischemic attacks
    c. Cerebral venous thrombosis
    d. Acute hemorrhagic cerebral infarction

33. Which of the following statements is correct concerning management of neurologic disease and pregnancy?
- a. Disease modifying therapy for multiple sclerosis should not be interrupted for pregnancy or lactation
- b. In a woman with a known cerebral arteriovenous malformation (AVM), pregnancy should be delayed until the lesion can be definitively treated
- c. A woman with a known cerebral arteriovenous malformation should not deliver her baby vaginally under any circumstances
- d. Women with myasthenia gravis should not take anticholinesterase medications during pregnancy

34. What is the most accurate way to educate a patient contemplating surgery for an unruptured intracerebral arteriovenous malformation (AVM) about his risk of hemorrhage if the lesion is not treated?
- a. The patient should be reassured, because the risk of hemorrhage is only 2%-4% per year
- b. Patients with particularly large AVMs should not be reassured, because they have a higher than average risk of bleeding
- c. The patient should understand that even though there is a substantial lifetime risk of hemorrhage, the risk of death with hemorrhage is low
- d. The patient should understand that although the risk of hemorrhage is low during any given year, the cumulative lifetime risk of hemorrhage is well over 50%

35. Which of the following best characterizes postoperative nursing management of the patient who has just undergone surgical treatment for an intracerebral arteriovenous malformation (AVM)?
- a. Mild systemic hypotension is permissible to avoid hemorrhage
- b. Mild systemic hypertension is permissible to avoid bleeding due to vasospasm
- c. Fluids should be relatively restricted to avoid cerebral venous hypertension and resulting increases in intracranial pressure
- d. Fluids should be relatively restricted because of the high likelihood of developing the syndrome of inappropriate ADH (SIADH)

36. The MOST important element of prevention of future strokes for the patient who has had lacunar infarcts is:
- a. Careful glucose control with diet, supplemented by hypoglycemic agents if necessary
- b. Management of hypertension
- c. Anticoagulation
- d. Anti-platelet drugs

37. A 25 year-old man is admitted to the hospital with severe throbbing right-sided headache and transient ipsilateral monocular blindness 3 days after an automobile accident in which he sustained no blunt trauma. Imaging studies have been ordered and are pending. Periodic nursing assessments should be particularly alert for:
    a. Swallowing problems and difficulty handling oral secretions
    b. Aphasia
    c. Partial Horner's syndrome
    d. Spatial neglect

38. A 23 year-old woman with a diagnosis of hemifacial spasm has had no benefit from decompression surgery. In fact, at surgery, no aberrant blood vessel was found in the vicinity of cranial nerve VII. She refuses anticonvulsant medication because she would like to become pregnant. The next step in her management should be:
    a. A new MRI scan, with double gadolinium and FLAIR sequences
    b. Psychiatric consultation and behavior management, including relaxation techniques
    c. Botulinum toxin
    d. Dental consultation to look for intraoral pathology that could be stimulating the unwanted movements

39. A patient with acute intracerebral hemorrhage has remained hypertensive, developed papillary edema, and now is becoming unresponsive. She has no respiratory problems, and her family is questioning preparations for endotracheal intubation. What is the most appropriate way to counsel the family?
    a. Tell the family that continued increased intracranial pressure puts her at risk for compression of her medullary respiratory center, and it is better to do a controlled elective intubation now than to intubate her on an emergency basis after respirations are compromised
    b. Initiate a medical ethics consultation
    c. Explain that the patient's increased intracranial pressure has reached a crisis level, putting the patient at risk for fatal pressure on her brainstem, and artificially inducing her to breathe rapidly can reduce the pressure inside her head by reducing the carbon dioxide concentration in her blood
    d. Prepare the family for the fact that the patient will remain intubated for at least several days, and ask for a speech therapy consultation to help the patient and family find a way to communicate during the period of intubation

40. A patient has hemineglect syndrome following a nondominant parietal lobe stroke. The MOST effective strategy is to:

    a. Approach the patient on the unaffected side of the body. If you must approach on the affected side, help the patient to turn his head toward you.

    b. Approach the patient on the affected side of the body as frequently as possible to help him to begin to pay attention to it again.

    c. Stimulate the affected side of the body frequently to flood the dysfunctional cerebral hemisphere with neural input.

    d. Request magnetic stimulation of the normal hemisphere to dampen its disproportionate activity so that the output from the damaged hemisphere is not overwhelmed.

41. Which of the following is the MOST appropriate nutritional supplement for a patient with multiple sclerosis and for his children?

    a. Vitamin C

    b. Vitamin B12

    c. Vitamin D

    d. Vitamin E

42. The best time to initiate range of motion (ROM) exercises following hemiplegic stroke is:

    a. At the onset of spasticity

    b. At the onset of synergy

    c. When fractures and other medical contraindications have been ruled out

    d. When the patient is conscious and motivated

43. Which of the following is a correct statement concerning the Bobath neurodevelopment approach to rehabilitation following hemiplegic stroke?

    a. The emphasis is on re-establishing normal movement patterns through having the patient experience the sensations of normal movement

    b. The emphasis is on muscle strengthening

    c. The emphasis is on overall conditioning, including cardiopulmonary fitness

    d. The emphasis is on adapting to new postures and patterns of movement imposed by the neurologic injury rather than on forcing the patient to try to recapture pre-stroke patterns of movement that are no longer possible

44. A fully conscious hemiplegic stroke patient should transfer from chair to bed by:

    a. Orienting the chair at an angle to the bed with the patient's affected side closest to the bed

    b. Orienting the chair at an angle to the bed with the patient's unaffected side closest to the bed

    c. Orienting the chair directly facing the bed

    d. Orienting the chair parallel to the bed with the patient's unaffected side closest to the bed

45. To prevent aspiration, which of the following precautions should be taken in caring for a patient who has had a brainstem stroke?
   a. Do not offer food or liquid until the patient has had normal barium swallow with videofluoroscopy
   b. Even when normal swallowing has been demonstrated, offer liquids first before attempting solids
   c. For hemiparetic or hemiplegic patients, place food in the mouth on the affected side to promote return of normal motor function
   d. Do not offer food or liquid until you have determined that the patient's gag reflex and swallowing reflex are intact

46. The MOST appropriate way to differentiate between an ischemic stroke and a hemorrhagic stroke is:
   a. Non-contrast CT scan of the brain
   b. CT scan of the brain without and with contrast
   c. MRI scan of the brain
   d. Lumbar puncture

47. In the setting of acute stroke, the BEST drug for intravenous control of hypertension is:
   a. Nitroprusside
   b. Furosemide
   c. Nimodipine
   d. Labetalol

48. The most common route by which infective agents enter the central nervous system is:
   a. Direct entry via skull injury
   b. Hematogenous spread
   c. Direct spread of adjacent infection involving the bones of the face, skull, or spine
   d. Contamination of surgical instruments or transplanted tissues, such as corneal grafts or dural patches

49. The pathogen most commonly responsible for bacterial meningitis in adolescents and young adults is:
   a. Group B Streptococcus
   b. Listeria monocytogenes
   c. Haemophilus influenzae
   d. Neisseria meningitides

50. The MOST COMMON source of infection leading to brain abscesses is
   a. Direct CNS invasion from otitis media and mastoiditis
   b. Sinusitis
   c. Hematogenous spread from distant infected sites, such as pneumonia, lung abscess, or bacterial endocarditis
   d. Accidental trauma and surgical injury

51. In which group is the incidence of intracranial hemorrhage greatest?
    a. Patients with intracranial aneurysms under 10 mm in diameter and no prior history of subarachnoid hemorrhage
    b. Patients with intracranial aneurysms greater than 10 mm in diameter and no prior history of subarachnoid hemorrhage
    c. Patients with unruptured intracerebral arteriovenous malformations
    d. Patients with carotid cavernous fistulas

52. In a patient with a negative non-contrast CT scan of the brain, the most reliable laboratory indicator of recent subarachnoid hemorrhage (SAH) is:
    a. A positive MRI scan of the brain
    b. Spectrophotometrically detected xanthochromia of the cerebrospinal fluid (CSF) obtained by lumbar puncture
    c. A positive contrast-enhanced CT scan of the brain
    d. Red blood cells in the cerebrospinal fluid (CSF) obtained by lumbar puncture

53. The underlying pathologic process in most lacunar infarcts is:
    a. Lipohyalinosis leading to microatheroma and thrombosis
    b. Cardioembolism
    c. Microhemorrhage
    d. Vascular malformation

54. The principal risk factor for lacunar infarct is
    a. Cigarette smoking
    b. Hyperlipidemia of any kind, including hypercholesterolemia
    c. Advanced age
    d. Hypertension

55. A patient has been all but disabled by daily migraines which have become unresponsive to any type of pain medication. Pharmacologic prophylaxis of her chronic daily headache is unlikely to be effective unless:
    a. The patient learns techniques of stress management
    b. The patient identifies her dietary triggers and eliminates them
    c. The patient is assisted to discontinue her pattern of daily analgesic use
    d. She adheres to a program of postural improvement and stretching exercises

56. Pain receptors are present in all of the following tissues EXCEPT:
    a. Brain parenchyma
    b. Periosteum of the skull
    c. Meninges
    d. Adventitia of the extracranial arteries

57. The MOST effective form of pharmacologic treatment for acute migraine once it has become moderately severe or severe is:
   a. A tricyclic antidepressant
   b. A beta-blocker
   c. A triptan or an ergot alkaloid
   d. Divalproex sodium

58. 100% oxygen via a non-rebreathing face mask at 7-10 L/min is effective acute treatment for what class of headache in approximately 60% of cases?
   a. Classic migraine
   b. Cluster headache
   c. Paroxysmal hemicrania
   d. Coital headache

59. In a 60 year-old female patient with dull headache and superimposed ice pick sensations on the scalp, jaw claudication, and elevated erythrocyte sedimentation rate (ESR,) the most important diagnostic test is:
   a. Lumbar puncture
   b. MRI scan of the brain without and with gadolinium
   c. Temporal artery biopsy
   d. Cerebral angiogram

60. For which class of headache does cigarette smoking constitute an insurmountable obstacle to pharmacologic prophylaxis?
   a. Common migraine
   b. Tension-type headache
   c. Migraine with aura
   d. Cluster headache

61. Which of the following is a correct statement about cerebrospinal fluid (CSF) leak due to a basal skull fracture?
   a. Prophylactic use of antibiotics is mandatory to prevent bacterial meningitis.
   b. Most CSF leaks persist for a matter of months, and patients should expect some CSF rhinorrhea for this period.
   c. CSF leak is a relatively infrequent complication of basal skull fracture, because abundant connective tissue cushions the dura from the bones at the base of the skull.
   d. A potential complication of basal skull fracture with CSF leak is trapping of portions of the frontal meninges between the fracture edges with a persistent CSF leak requiring surgical intervention.

62. A 6 year-old patient who has fallen and sustained closed head trauma has evidence of a nondisplaced right temporal skull fracture traversing the course of the middle meningeal artery. After an hour of lucidity and a normal neurologic examination, he complains of headache and develops hemiparesis. The next step in the evaluation should be:
   a. A non-contrast CT scan of the brain to look for evidence of an epidural hematoma
   b. A lumbar puncture to look for early evidence of central nervous system infection in the face of a likely dural tear
   c. A lumbar puncture to look for evidence of subarachnoid hemorrhage
   d. An EEG to look for a seizure focus, as the fall itself is unexplained

63. Most subdural hematomas arise from:
   a. Arterial bleeding from an intracranial artery directly injured by a fragment of skull
   b. Venous bleeding from torn bridging veins over the convexities of the brain
   c. Cerebral contusions
   d. Trauma superimposed upon an underlying coagulopathy

64. The diagnosis of mild diffuse axonal injury (DAI) following acceleration/deceleration injury is made:
   a. By noting multiple small hemorrhagic lesions on MRI
   b. By noting diffuse cerebral edema on CT scan
   c. By noting bifrontal slowing on EEG
   d. By noting the characteristic clinical features of coma of under 24 hours duration and no visible traumatic lesion on CT scan

65. A patient with traumatic brain injury has a Glasgow Coma Score of 8 and is intubated in the field because of cardiopulmonary arrest. While enroute to the hospital, the PRIMARY goal of ventilator management is:
   a. Inducing hypocapnia
   b. Preventing hypoxia
   c. Avoiding oxygen toxicity
   d. Normalizing intracranial pressure

66. A patient about to leave the ICU following a week of stabilization after traumatic brain injury develops hypertension, tachycardia, tachypnea, and fever. A thorough work-up produces no evidence of infection. Intervention at this point is MOST likely to include which of the following?
   a. Intravenous morphine sulfate
   b. Ventriculostomy for cerebrospinal fluid drainage
   c. Intravenous insulin
   d. Electroencephalogram

67. On the third day following traumatic brain injury, a patient develops an oval pupil on one side. This is MOST likely to be a sign of:
   a. Optic nerve injury
   b. Impending transtentorial herniation
   c. Autonomic dysfunction syndrome
   d. Carotid-cavernous fistula

68. The best way to accomplish external draining of cerebrospinal fluid through an external ventricular drain is:
   a. Drain several ml of fluid over a period of no longer than one minute, and then promptly close the drain
   b. Drain as much fluid as necessary to keep intracranial pressure (ICP) below 15 mm Hg
   c. Drain a few minidrops per minute, and close the drain after 5 minutes or less
   d. Drain continuously, keeping the drain open for as long as necessary until intracranial pressure stabilizes

69. One should never suction the airway through the nose in the presence of:
   a. A pituitary adenoma
   b. A carotid-cavernous fistula
   c. Increased intracranial pressure
   d. A basal skull fracture

70. Following spinal injury, a patient is delivered to the emergency department in a hard cervical collar on a backboard. It is the nurse's role to:
   a. Remove the backboard when spine X-rays have been completed and serious injury excluded
   b. Keep track of how long the patient has been on the board and inform the rest of the team
   c. Turn the patient carefully from time to time and then resume immobilization
   d. Transfer the patient to a backboard belonging to the emergency department

71. As soon as a spinal cord injured patient arrives in the emergency department, bladder management is initiated by:
   a. Initiating intermittent catheterization
   b. Placing an indwelling urinary catheter
   c. Asking the patient if he can void
   d. Starting antibiotics to prevent urinary tract infection

72. When a spinal cord injured patient arrives in the emergency department, management of the gastrointestinal system in initiated by:
   a. Evaluating masticatory function and swallowing
   b. Establishing venous access for total parenteral nutrition
   c. Withholding food until the patient can safely sit up to eat
   d. Inserting a nasogastric tube set to low intermittent suction

73. A patient with spinal cord injury suddenly complains of a severe pounding headache and is noted to be sweating profusely above the level of his cord lesion, with cool, dry, pale skin below the level of the lesion Blood pressure is 200/110, and pulse is 50. The organ system that should be assessed FIRST is:
    a. The cardiovascular system
    b. The nervous system
    c. The urinary system
    d. The gastrointestinal system

74. The MOST common cause of radial nerve injury is:
    a. A fractured humerus
    b. A fractured radius
    c. A fractured ulna
    d. Shoulder dislocation

75. A woman in the third trimester of pregnancy has been sleeping in her chair because of heartburn, and she begins to wake up every night because of pain in her forearms. She has positive Tinel's and Phalen's signs bilaterally. Her best treatment option at this point is:
    a. Surgical decompression of the carpal tunnel on the non-dominant side, followed by surgical decompression of the dominant side after she has healed from the first surgery
    b. Changing her sleep position so that her upper arms do not drape over the arms of her chair
    c. Corticosteroid injections into the carpal tunnel
    d. Wrist splints and rehabilitation modalities

76. All of the following are risk factors for chronic subdural hematoma (SDH) EXCEPT:
    a. Female sex
    b. Age over 50 years
    c. Alcoholism
    d. Trauma

77. A patient with traumatic brain injury regains consciousness after several days in intensive care. As he recovers, it becomes clear that he has unilateral foot drop, and he is complaining of burning pain over the top of the foot on the same side. This complication could have been avoided by:
    a. Avoiding excessive flexion at the hip during the period when he was immobilized
    b. Avoiding pressure to the back of his knee during the period when he was immobilized
    c. Providing passive range of motion exercises during the period when he was immobilized
    d. Providing splints to keep the feet in dorsiflexion during the period when he was immobilized

78. The main difference between a subdural hematoma and a subdural hygroma is:
    a. A subdural hygroma is usually asymptomatic
    b. A subdural hygroma is usually bilateral
    c. A subdural hygroma is derived from arterial blood
    d. A subdural hygroma is composed of cerebrospinal fluid

79. Following spinal cord injury, the primary goal of a maintenance bowel management program is to:
   a. Avoid the use of laxatives
   b. Allow the patient to have a soft, formed bowel movement every 1 to 3 days
   c. Prevent Valsalva's maneuver, because it can trigger autonomic dysreflexia (AD)
   d. Insure that the patient defecates at the same time every day

80. A patient known to be schizophrenic is brought to the emergency room in status epilepticus and has a serum sodium concentration of 109 mEq/L. The seizures stop when he has received intravenous phenytoin. The approach to correcting the serum sodium should be:
   a. Rapid normalization with hypertonic saline to remove the underlying cause of the seizures
   b. Slow normalization with demeclocycline to address the underlying cause of the hyponatremia
   c. Slow normalization with water restriction to avoid abrupt fluid shifts
   d. Slow normalization with hypertonic saline and furosemide to avoid central pontine myelinolysis

81. A patient who has been admitted following an automobile accident with trauma to multiple parts of the body is noted to have severe sharp pain on passive hip flexion. This should raise suspicion of:
   a. Meningeal irritation
   b. Fractured hip
   c. Herniated nucleus pulposus in the lumbar spine
   d. Fractured pelvis

82. Following spinal cord injury, the MOST important reason to monitor the neurologic examination at intervals of 2 hours or less is to:
   a. Detect evidence of peripheral nerve injury that escaped early notice because it was masked by the central nervous system lesion
   b. Detect evidence of late-developing brain dysfunction due to another injury, such as delayed accumulation of an epidural hematoma
   c. Detect evidence of early recovery, which has important prognostic implications
   d. Detect evidence of ascending spinal cord edema

83. The MOST common cause of low back pain in middle-aged individuals is:
   a. Herniated nucleus pulposus at L5/S1
   b. Lumbar spinal stenosis
   c. Lumbar spondylolysis
   d. Lumbar strain

84. The one alternative approach that has been shown to be effective in reducing symptoms of carpal tunnel syndrome is:
    a. Yoga
    b. Chiropractic
    c. Acupuncture
    d. Relaxation techniques

85. Which of the following is NOT a risk factor for Erb's palsy?
    a. Gestational diabetes in the mother
    b. Premature delivery
    c. Shoulder dystocia
    d. Pharmacologic induction or acceleration of labor

86. The MOST important element of education for parents of a baby with Erb's palsy prior to discharge from the hospital or labor facility is:
    a. Instruction in passive range of motion exercises (ROM) for the affected arm
    b. Referral to a surgeon for brachial plexus exploration and nerve grafting
    c. Instruction to strongly consider elective Caesarian section for subsequent children
    d. Conference with the hospital's risk management department

87. A patient discharged to home after hospitalization for multiple traumas that included a frontal bone fracture should receive education to avoid:
    a. Choking on food
    b. Aspiration of food
    c. Vitamin deficiencies
    d. Food poisoning

88. The PRIMARY purpose of otoscopic examination of the unconscious patient who is brought to the emergency room without a diagnosis is:
    a. To look for hemotympanum or otorrhea
    b. To look for a perimeningeal site of infection
    c. To look for signs of vestibular dysfunction
    d. To look for Battle's sign

89. Which of the following is NOT a recommended treatment for patients with increased intracranial pressure following traumatic brain injury?
    a. Barbiturates
    b. Hyperventilation
    c. Hypertonic saline
    d. Glucocorticoids

90. Intravenous phenytoin should not be given any faster than 50 mg/min because of the risks of:
   a. Hypotension and cardiac arrhythmia
   b. Allergic reaction
   c. Vein injury
   d. Tissue damage in the event of extravasation

91. It is advisable to avoid glucose-containing intravenous fluids for patients with traumatic brain injury (TBI) because glucose can contribute to:
   a. Neurotoxic acidosis
   b. Cerebral edema
   c. Hyponatremia
   d. Hypokalemia

92. It is important to explain to young epilepsy patients and their families that the MOST compelling reason for monitoring serum anticonvulsant levels in a young person with epilepsy is that:
   a. Children, and especially adolescents, are frequently noncompliant with prescribed medications
   b. Many children outgrow their epilepsy
   c. Even in the absence of apparent side effects, such as drowsiness, anticonvulsant drugs at excessive serum concentrations can inhibit normal growth and development
   d. Even with good compliance, drug levels will change as children grow

93. Intravenous phenytoin should be administered in a fluid that is free of:
   a. Potassium
   b. Thiamine
   c. Dextrose
   d. Sodium

94. A patient is brought to the emergency room after having been found unconscious. He appears pale and cachectic and may have alcohol on his breath. As soon as intravenous access is established, this patient should receive:
   a. 10% dextrose in water intravenously
   b. 5% dextrose in normal saline intravenously
   c. Thiamine intramuscularly
   d. Vitamin B12 intramuscularly

95. A healthy 3rd-grader with apparent high intelligence has been underperforming in school ever since first grade. She often fails to follow directions, although she seems well motivated. There have been multiple parent-teacher conferences to address this. Eventually, the teacher notices a brief staring spell during which the child does not respond to her name, and a medical consultation ensues. The electroencephalogram (EEG) is MOST likely to show:
   a. A seizure focus in the mesial temporal lobe
   b. Generalized 3-Hz spike-wave complexes
   c. Bilateral polyspikes
   d. Periodic lateralized epileptiform discharges

96. Of the following, the MOST common reason that people with multiple sclerosis (MS) stop working is:
   a. Cognitive impairment
   b. Workplace discrimination
   c. Chronic pain
   d. Incontinence

97. The goal of surgical therapy for most primary malignant brain tumors is:
   a. Cure
   b. Prevention of distant metastases
   c. Relieving increased intracranial pressure
   d. Safe removal of as much viable tumor as possible without causing unacceptable neurologic deficits

98. A disadvantage of gamma-knife treatment compared with other treatment modalities for malignant brain tumors is that:
   a. It fails to eliminate undetected malignant cells that have infiltrated into surrounding normal tissue
   b. It causes too much damage to surrounding normal tissue
   c. It causes too much cerebral edema
   d. It is not curative

99. In general, primary malignant brain tumors are relatively unresponsive to chemotherapy. A notable exception to this rule is a particular subset of:
   a. Astrocytoma
   b. Craniopharyngioma
   c. Ependymoma
   d. Oligodendroglioma

100. The incidence of medulloblastoma:
   a. Increases with age
   b. Decreases with age
   c. Peaks in the fifth decade
   d. Has a bimodal distribution, with peaks in the third and fifth decades

101. Many histologically benign brain tumors prove to be fatal because:
   a. They undergo malignant transformation
   b. They are in locations that are surgically inaccessible, so they continue to grow
   c. They constitute a seizure focus, and the patient succumbs in status epilepticus
   d. They occlude the ventricular system, causing increased intracranial pressure

102. Which of the following is NOT a brain tumor of neuroepithelial origin?
    a. Astrocytoma
    b. Oligodendroglioma
    c. Ependymoma
    d. Pituitary adenoma

103. The goals of surgical treatment of acoustic neuroma are to:
    a. Remove the tumor and restore hearing
    b. Remove the tumor and prevent facial paralysis
    c. Remove the tumor and prevent metastasis
    d. Reduce the size of the tumor and slow its growth

104. The most common location of a central nervous system hemangioblastoma is:
    a. The posterior fossa
    b. The spinal cord
    c. The cerebral hemispheres
    d. The optic nerves

105. A patient presents with ataxia and headache. MRI scan reveals an enhancing cerebellar lesion with surrounding edema, and a complete blood count shows elevated red cell count and hematocrit. Further work-up reveals a tumor in one adrenal gland. Family members of this patient should have:
    a. MRI scan of the brain
    b. MRI scan of the abdomen to examine the kidneys and adrenal glands
    c. Genetic testing
    d. Complete blood count

106. A patient taking methotrexate for treatment of primary central nervous system lymphoma should avoid aspirin and nonsteroidal anti-inflammatory agents (NSAIDs) because they:
    a. Reduce serum concentration of methotrexate, potentially rendering the drug ineffective
    b. Reduce serum half-life of methotrexate, potentially rendering the drug ineffective
    c. Increase the serum concentration of methotrexate, thus increasing the already substantial risk of toxicity
    d. Increase the serum concentration of methotrexate and prolong its serum half-life, thus increasing the already substantial risk of toxicity

107. The MOST significant risk factor for primary central nervous system lymphoma is:
    a. Immunosuppression of any kind
    b. Female gender
    c. Age over 60
    d. Multiple sexual partners

108. The family of a child who has recently been diagnosed with neurofibromatosis is seeking genetic information and counseling. While a genetics consultation is pending, you can tell them that:
    a.The disorder is inherited in an autosomal recessive fashion
    b. The disorder is inherited in a sex-linked fashion
    c. The disorder is usually not inherited
    d. The disorder is inherited in an autosomal dominant fashion, but as many as one-third of cases occur as spontaneous mutations

109. The tumors that occur in von-Hippel Lindau disease are:
    a. Hemangiomas
    b. Schwannomas
    c. Gliomas
    d. Meningiomas

110. The only fully established risk factor for meningioma is:
    a. Cigarette smoking
    b. Radiation exposure
    c. Asbestos exposure
    d. Pesticide exposure

111. A patient with a known pituitary adenoma experiences the abrupt onset of headache and visual loss. The most likely approach will be:
    a. Radiation therapy
    b. Minimally invasive surgery
    c. Ventriculostomy
    d. Hyperventilation

112. Prior to undergoing endoscopic surgery to remove a pituitary adenoma, a patient must have:
    a. Adequate thyroid hormone and glucocorticoid levels
    b. A normal hematocrit
    c. Intact visual fields
    d. Normal prolactin level

113. The tumor most likely to present with bitemporal hemianopia is:
    a. Carcinoma of the lung metastatic to both occipital lobes
    b. Carcinoma of the breast metastatic to both temporal lobes
    c. Pituitary adenoma
    d. Astrocytoma of the optic nerve

114. Surgical treatment is indicated for cholesteatoma:
    a. When it leads to central nervous system infection, such as meningitis
    b. Whenever it is diagnosed
    c. When it leads to impaired hearing
    d. When it leads to infection in the mastoid air cells

115. The GREATEST improvement in survival rates in recent years of patients with cancers metastatic to the brain is attributable to:
    a. Whole brain radiation therapy
    b. Focal brain surgery
    c. Improved chemotherapy delivery systems
    d. Radiosurgery

116. First-line therapy for nearly all intramedullary spinal tumors is:
    a. Surgical resection
    b. Radiation therapy
    c. Chemotherapy
    d. Watchful waiting

117. Chemotherapy for the treatment of primary intramedullary spinal cord tumors is considered to be:
    a. An important adjunct to surgical excision
    b. An important adjunct to radiation therapy
    c. Contraindicated
    d. Experimental

118. During surgery for spinal cord tumors, general anesthesia with halogenated volatile anesthetics is not advised because:
    a. They may lead to decreased spinal cord perfusion and resulting spinal cord infarction
    b. They interfere with somatosensory evoked potentials
    c. Their metabolism is inhibited by nitric oxide (NO)
    d. They can lead to cardiac arrhythmias

119. A NEGATIVE prognostic factor for complete neurologic recovery following surgery for a spinal cord tumor is:
    a. Severe neurologic deficit prior to surgery
    b. Presence of a syrinx
    c Female sex
    d. Tumor involving the lumbar cord

120. The most common route of metastasis of malignant tumors from other organs to the central nervous system is:
    a. Via the lymphatic system
    b. Direct penetration from adjacent structures
    c. Via the blood circulation
    d. Via the spinal fluid

121. The evidence-based standard of care for pharmacologic management of Bell's palsy is:
    a. Antiviral medication alone
    b. Steroid medication alone
    c. Antiviral medication and steroids combined
    d. Interferon beta alone

122. Each of the following is a potential symptom of a Chiari malformation EXCEPT:
    a. Headache
    b. Impaired fine motor coordination in the hands
    c. Numbness and tingling in the hands and feet
    d. Seizures

123. A comprehensive review of over 35,000 births by the National Institute of Neurologic Disorders and Stroke (NINDS) during the 1980s showed that complications of childbirth accounted for what percentage of cases of cerebral palsy?
    a. 90% or more
    b. 75%
    c. 50%
    d. 10% or less

124. The FIRST line of therapy to treat spasticity associated with cerebral palsy is:
    a. Physical therapy
    b. Oral medication, such as baclofen or tizanidine
    c. Intramuscular botulinum toxin
    d. Intrathecal baclofen

125. All of the following are risk factors for spina bifida EXCEPT:
    a. Pre-pregnancy maternal obesity
    b. Maternal diabetes
    c. Birth trauma
    d. Maternal folic acid deficiency

126. Spina bifida is frequently associated with:
    a. Myelomeningocele
    b. Anencephaly
    c. Epilepsy
    d. Cerebral palsy

127. Elevated maternal serum alpha-fetoprotein is a marker for:
    a. Down's syndrome
    b. Spina bifida
    c. Cerebral palsy
    d. Chiari malformation

128. The natural history of untreated syringomyelia is:
    a. Usually benign, with stabilization and minimal disability
    b. Characterized by exacerbations and remissions
    c. Usually rapidly progressive, with significant disability within 2 years of diagnosis
    d. Usually slowly progressive, with slow accumulation of neurologic deficits over many years

129. Treating spasticity in patients with syringomyelia:
    a. Should be balanced so as not to inadvertently increase bladder dysfunction
    b. Should be balanced so as not to inadvertently increase pain
    c. Should be balanced so as not to inadvertently increase weakness
    d. Should be balanced so as not to inadvertently decrease pain and temperature sensation

130. The frontotemporal dementias are characterized by:
    a. Impaired language function out of proportion to other cognitive deficits
    b. Impaired capacity to plan and carry out complex tasks out of proportion to other cognitive deficits
    c. Impaired recent memory out of proportion to other cognitive deficits
    d. Impaired spatial orientation out of proportion to other cognitive deficits

131. Patients taking huperzine A (Chinese club moss) to treat Alzheimer's Disease should not concurrently take:
    a. Prescription cholinesterase inhibitors
    b. Prescription memantine
    c. Vitamin E
    d. Ginkgo biloba

132. Cholinesterase inhibitors:
    a. Reverse the cognitive deficits of 50% of patients with Alzheimer's disease
    b. Delay worsening of symptoms for 6 to 12 months for about 50% of patients with Alzheimer's disease
    c. Decrease levels of acetylcholine in critical parts of the brain
    d. Should not be given concurrently with vitamin E

133. The BEST strategy to insure that a patient in the middle stages of Alzheimer's Disease executes complex instructions correctly is to:
    a. Provide a written list of steps to be taken in numbered order, using large print
    b. Provide verbal and nonverbal cues simultaneously
    c. Speak loudly and clearly to gain the patient's attention and confidence
    d. Leave object cues in the environment

134. Which is the best way to begin lunch with a patient with Alzheimer's Disease?
    a. "What would you like to eat?"
    b. "I ordered a hamburger for you."
    c. "Did you like yesterday's lunch?"
    d. "Would you like the pasta or the tuna sandwich?"

135. The BEST response when a patient with Alzheimer's Disease experiences hallucinations or delusions is:
    a. Deny the reality of the experience
    b. Affirm the reality of the experience
    c. Provide antipsychotic medication
    d. Take all necessary steps to assure the patient's safety and reassure the patient

136. A predisposition to generalized seizures occurs in patients with:
    a. Advanced multiple sclerosis
    b. Stage 3 Alzheimer's disease
    c. Advanced Parkinson's disease
    d. Normal pressure hydrocephalus

137. A patient presenting with impaired memory, broad-based magnetic gait and urinary incontinence to which he is indifferent is most likely to respond to:
    a. Ventriculoperitoneal shunt
    b. Donepezil
    c. Carbidopa/levodopa
    d. Antidepressant medication

138. Dementia with a step-wise clinical progression is most likely to be due to:
    a. Alzheimer's Disease
    b. Normal pressure hydrocephalus
    c. Depression
    d. Multiple silent cerebral infarctions

139. The MOST significant risk factor for the development of pseudotumor cerebri is:
    a. Obesity
    b. Cigarette smoking
    c. Oral contraceptives
    d. Lyme disease

140. The most serious complication of pseudotumor cerebri is:
    a. Herniation of the cerebellar tonsils through the foramen magnum
    b. Deafness
    c. Blindness
    d. Status epilepticus

141. Tremor that occurs most prominently whenever the hands are in use, as opposed to when the hands are at rest most likely represents:
    a. Medication toxicity
    b. Cerebellar dysfunction
    c. Parkinson's Disease
    d. Benign essential tremor

142. A person over the age of 65 years presenting with tremor, rigidity, and bradykinesia most likely has:
   a. Parkinson's Disease
   b. Benign essential tremor
   c. Huntington's Disease
   d. Normal pressure hydrocephalus

143. Levodopa is used instead of dopamine itself to treat symptoms of Parkinson's Disease because:
   a. Levodopa is more potent than dopamine
   b. Levodopa crosses the blood-brain barrier, and dopamine does not
   c. Levodopa can be given with carbidopa, and dopamine cannot
   d. Levodopa is not associated with side effects such as psychosis

144. The role of carbidopa in pharmacologic management of the symptoms of Parkinson's Disease is:
   a. To prolong the half-life of levodopa
   b. To elevate the serum concentration of levodopa
   c. To inhibit the enzyme dopa decarboxylase
   d. To smooth out the "on-off" phenomenon

145. Which is the dietary modification most likely to be needed eventually for a patient with Parkinson's disease?
   a. A very low-protein diet
   b. A low-calcium diet
   c. Soft foods and liquids only
   d. Coarsely ground foods and small, supervised feedings

146. The use of anticholinergic medications given to patients with Parkinson's Disease:
   a. Often reduces tremor and drooling
   b. Is intended to improve cognitive function
   c. Has a neuroprotective effect
   d. Is limited by diarrhea as a side-effect

147. Prior to deep brain stimulation for management of Parkinson's Disease (PD):
   a. PD medications are gradually tapered over a period of several days and then discontinued
   b. PD medications are continued without change
   c. The patient should undergo a supervised drug holiday
   d. PD medications are discontinued the night before surgery

148. The dietary supplement most appropriate for patients with Wilson's Disease is:
   a. Vitamin D
   b. Zinc acetate
   c. Folic acid
   d. Thiamine

149. The most prevalent focal dystonia is:
   a. Blepharospasm
   b. Torsion dystonia (dystonia musculorum deformans)
   c. Writer's cramp
   d. Torticollis

150. Dietary management of a patient with hypokalemic periodic paralysis includes:
   a. Avoidance of caffeine
   b. Avoidance of high-protein meals
   c. Avoidance of high-carbohydrate meals
   d. Calcium supplementation

151. The best approach to maximizing neurologic development for an infant with Down syndrome is:
   a. The ketogenic diet
   b. Early intervention with sensory, motor, and cognitive activities
   c. Proactive use of anticonvulsant medication
   d. A diet low in long-chain fatty acids, supplemented by glyceryl trioleate and glyceryl trierucate

152. Individuals with Down syndrome have the GREATEST increased risk of:
   a. Dementia
   b. Psychosis
   c. Generalized anxiety disorder
   d. Epilepsy

153. A young woman with Down syndrome and her family wonder about the likelihood of her offspring having Down syndrome if she becomes pregnant. What should you tell them?
   a. Her offspring will have Down syndrome.
   b. She has the same risk of having a child with Down syndrome as any other woman in her age group.
   c. She has a 35-50% risk of having a child with Down syndrome or another developmental disorder.
   d. Women with Down syndrome do not become pregnant.

154. A child with Down syndrome who has been progressing well in school begins to have trouble paying attention in class and fails to learn new material without a great deal of repetition, but does not lose previously acquired cognitive skills. The diagnostic test MOST likely to provide a relevant diagnosis is:
   a. Electroencephalogram
   b. Electrocardiogram
   c. Echocardiography
   d. Polysomnography

155. A baby with Down syndrome is MOST likely to need:
    a. A feeding tube
    b. Manual support of the chin and throat during breast feeding
    c. A gluten-free formula
    d. Thyroid hormone supplementation

156. A patient who takes a sustained-release opioid medication on a time contingent schedule to treat chronic pain should be educated to expect to experience all of the following EXCEPT:
    a. Dependence
    b. Tolerance
    c. Addiction
    d. Constipation

157. Tolerance to opioid medication is wholly or partially preventable by:
    a. Dextromethorphan
    b. Naloxone
    c. Naltrexone
    d. Methadone

158. Neuropathic pain is usually:
    a. Most severe in the morning
    b. Bimodal, with peaks in the morning and again in the evening
    c. Most severe in the evening
    d. Lacking in any diurnal pattern

159. A symmetric, bilateral distribution of sensory and motor deficits, beginning distally and progressing proximally most likely represents:
    a. Mononeuropathy multiplex
    b. Mononeuropathy simplex
    c. Paraneoplastic syndrome
    d. Diabetic peripheral polyneuropathy

160. A patient being issued crutches for any reason should be instructed in their correct use in order to avoid:
    a. Median nerve entrapment injury
    b. Brachial plexus stretch injury
    c. Radial nerve entrapment injury
    d. Ulnar nerve entrapment injury

161. The family of a child with adrenoleukodystrophy (ALD) is seeking genetic counseling. Along with the requested referral, the family can be told that the inheritance of adrenoleukodystrophy is:
    a. Nearly always X-linked recessive
    b. Nearly always autosomal dominant
    c. Nearly always autosomal recessive
    d. Nearly always polygenic

162. Patients with adrenoleukodystrophy lack:
    a. An enzyme that breaks down glycogen
    b. The enzyme acid alpha-glucosidase
    c. The enzyme hexosaminidase
    d. An enzyme that breaks down very long chain fatty acids

163. Women are three times more likely than men to develop:
    a. Parkinson's Disease
    b. Adult-onset epilepsy
    c. Carpal tunnel syndrome
    d. Alcoholism

164. The MOST common neurologic manifestation of HIV disease is:
    a. AIDS encephalopathy
    b. Peripheral neuropathy
    c. Myelopathy
    d. Opportunistic infections of the central nervous system

165. A patient with HIV disease is taking isoniazid (INH), rifampin (RIF), ethambutol (EMB) and pyrazinamide (PZA.) The nutritional supplement MOST important to include in this patient's regimen is:
    a. Pyridoxine (vitamin B6)
    b. Vitamin D
    c. Vitamin E
    d. Vitamin B12

166. When children with attention deficit hyperactivity disorder (ADHD) enter their teenage years:
    a. Most will outgrow their symptoms
    b. Their risk of developing tic disorders increases
    c. Their risk of automobile accidents is greater than the risk of other teens
    d. They should not change their dose of stimulant medication

167. Restless leg syndrome (RLS):
    a. Affects mainly older adults
    b. Affects mainly pregnant women
    c. Affects mainly people with Parkinson's disease
    d. Affects people of all ages

168. The BEST approach to pharmacologic management of symptoms of restless leg syndrome (RLS) is usually:
    a. Opioid medication at bedtime
    b. Tricyclic antidepressant medication at bedtime
    c. Cyclic deployment of various classes of medications
    d. Dopaminergic medication at bedtime

169. Multiple sclerosis patients treated with natalizumab (Tysabri) require intensive long-term monitoring because:
    a. They have a 1/1000 risk of developing progressive multifocal leukoencephalopathy
    b. They have a 4% risk of developing an allergic reaction
    c. They have a risk of serious depression
    d. They are likely to become non-compliant because of the need for frequent injections

170. The GREATEST risk factor for progressive multifocal leukoencephalopathy (PML) is:
    a. Multiple sclerosis
    b. Organ transplantation
    c. Leukemia
    d. AIDS

171. Fibromyalgia is fundamentally:
    a. A neurologic disorder
    b. A rheumatologic disorder
    c. A psychiatric disorder
    d. A form of malingering

172. At the onset of an attack of vertigo associated with Ménière's Disease, it is best to:
    a. Read or watch television for distraction
    b. Walk around, using external supports as needed
    c. Listen to music
    d. Lie down and rest until the attack has completely subsided

173. Individuals with Ménière's Disease are at increased risk for:
    a. Falls
    b. Accidents while driving vehicles or operating machinery
    c. Depression
    d. All of the above

174. BEFORE embarking on treatment with a time-contingent regimen of a sustained-release opioid medication for chronic non-cancer pain, it is essential to:
    a. Discontinue any short-acting opioids the patient has been taking
    b. Have the patient and doctor sign an agreement that specifies their mutual expectations and parameters of treatment
    c. Pretreat the patient with dextromethorphan
    d. Obtain consultation with a psychologist or psychiatrist

175. The MOST COMMON natural history of degenerative disc disease without radiculopathy in the lumbar spine is:
    a. Gradual, steady worsening of pain over time without other symptoms
    b. Relentless spread to adjacent discs
    c. Gradual improvement over time
    d. Gradual development of radiculopathy and/or instability over time

176. Low back pain due to degenerative lumbar disc disease is usually:
   a. Exacerbated by walking and/or running
   b. Exacerbated by sitting
   c. Exacerbated by lateral rotation
   d. Exacerbated by lying down

177. Spondylolisthesis in children is MOST OFTEN:
   a. Traumatic
   b. Congenital
   c. Pathological (e.g. secondary to tumor)
   d. Degenerative

178. Death due to multiple system atrophy is MOST often due to:
   a. Hypoperfusion
   b. Aspiration
   c. Central respiratory failure
   d. Malnutrition

179. Many patients with multiple system atrophy become overheated and are
at significant risk for heat stroke because:
   a. They fail to sweat
   b. They cannot take in adequate fluids because of their dysphagia
   c. They have a dominant gene that causes them to develop hypermetabolism and muscle
      contractures in response to certain stimuli
   d. Their peripheral capillaries cannot dilate adequately to regulate body temperature

180. Which of the following is NOT a risk factor for vertebral compression fracture?
   a. Female gender
   b. Osteoporosis
   c. Cigarette smoking
   d. Obesity

181. Back and leg pain caused by lumbar spinal stenosis usually:
   a. Worsens when the patient bends forward
   b. Worsens when the patient sits down
   c. Improves somewhat with walking uphill
   d. Improves somewhat with walking downhill

182. The primary risk factor for spinal stenosis is:
   a. Advancing age
   b. Male gender
   c. Cigarette smoking
   d. Multiple injuries

183. Untreated hydrocephalus in newborns:
   a. Usually resolves on its own
   b. Is not a grave concern because the fontanelles are open
   c. Is most likely to have a favorable outcome if associated with infection
   d. Has a 50-60% death rate overall

184. The general term for a document that gives directions concerning a person's health care in the event that he can no longer make decisions for himself is:
   a. Durable power of attorney for health care
   b. Advance directive
   c. Living will
   d. Health care proxy

185. The varicella-zoster vaccine (Zostavax) is recommended for:
   a. Adults over 60 years old who have never had chickenpox
   b. People of any age who have any condition that causes immunosuppression
   c. Immunologically intact adults over age 60 who have had chickenpox
   d. Adults over age 60 who have had zoster

186. Triptans should not be used to abort migraine headaches in patients who:
   a. Have hypertension or other risk factors for heart attack or stroke
   b. Have clotting disorders
   c. Have peptic ulcer disease
   d. Are immunosuppressed

187. The MOST effective strategy to date for limiting cognitive impairment in patients with multiple sclerosis (MS) is:
   a. Oral memantine
   b. Early intervention with disease-modifying agents
   c. Oral donepezil
   d. Oral l-amphetamine

188. Injection site reactions are LEAST frequently encountered by patients treating their multiple sclerosis with:
   a. Subcutaneous interferon beta-1a
   b. Subcutaneous interferon beta-1b
   c. Subcutaneous glatiramer acetate
   d. Intramuscular interferon beta-1a

189. A patient is in a persistent vegetative state following head trauma. In the year preceding her injury, she executed an advance directive that specified the types of medical interventions she would deem acceptable in this type of situation. Her family members find themselves in bitter conflict over the question of withdrawing life-sustaining medical interventions, and a hospital ethicist has been consulted to facilitate communications. Among the ethical considerations that pertain to this situation, the consideration that takes the GREATEST priority is:
  a. Beneficence
  b. Autonomy
  c. Justice
  d. Dignity

190. Brain death is characterized by:
  a. Coma or unresponsiveness
  b. Apnea
  c. Absence of brainstem reflexes
  d. All of the above

191. Zostavax is:
  a. A killed virus vaccine indicated for prevention of chickenpox
  b. A killed virus vaccine indicated for prevention of shingles
  c. A live attenuated virus vaccine indicated for prevention of herpes infections
  d. A live attenuated virus vaccine indicated for prevention of shingles

192. Sympathetic blockade can reduce the pain associated with:
  a. Trigeminal neuralgia
  b. Glossopharyngeal neuralgia
  c. Postherpetic neuralgia
  d. Occipital neuralgia

193. Spinal headaches are ALWAYS:
  a. Caused by cerebrospinal fluid (CSF) leak following lumbar puncture
  b. Caused by intracranial hypotension
  c. Relieved by a blood patch
  d. Relieved by aggressive hydration and caffeine

194. Patients with Huntington's Disease who develop symptoms during the early adult years often present with symptoms and signs that mimic:
  a. Parkinson's disease
  b. Multiple sclerosis
  c. Myasthenia gravis
  d. Alzheimer's Disease

195. If a person has one parent with Huntington's disease, his chance of also having Huntington's disease is:
    a. 100%
    b. 75%
    c. 50%
    d. 25%

196. Antibiotic treatment for neurosyphilis:
    a. Is contraindicated because the risk of Jarisch-Herxheimer reaction outweighs the benefit of treatment for patients who already have irreversible end-organ damage
    b. Should consist of intravenous aqueous crystalline Penicillin G every four hours for 10-14 days
    c. Should consist of 3 weekly doses of benzathine Penicillin G
    d. Should be combined with HAART (highly active antiretroviral therapy) because syphilis is so closely associated with HIV disease

197. When a woman known to have multiple sclerosis (MS) gives birth:
    a. She should not have epidural anesthesia because of the risk of producing an exacerbation.
    b. She should be advised to choose Caesarean section, especially if she has prominent motor weakness.
    c. A pediatrician should be present at the delivery because of the risk of respiratory compromise in the infant.
    d. Her choice of interventions for pain should be made based on the same obstetric considerations and personal preferences as for any other woman.

198. The BEST method for preventing subacute sclerosing panencephalitis (SSPE) is:
    a. Measles vaccination
    b. Intrathecal isoprinosine
    c. Oral isoprinosine
    d. Interferon alpha

199. Parents should be educated to understand that the BEST method for preventing Reye' syndrome is:
    a. Chickenpox vaccination
    b. Measles vaccination
    c. Avoiding salicylates in treating children with viral illnesses
    d. Avoiding acetaminophen in treating children with viral illnesses

200. Each year during flu season, there is public discussion of Guillain-Barré syndrome. Patients should be aware that the risk factor MOST strongly linked to development of Guillain-Barré syndrome (GBS) is:
    a. Immunization against seasonal influenza
    b. Immunization against novel recombinant influenza viruses
    c. Underlying abnormalities of myelin
    d. Antecedent bacterial or viral illness

201. The MOST practical system of communication that can be implemented by the nurse for a patient with locked-in syndrome is:
- a. A simple system of eye blinks and other eye movements to correlate with simple responses, such as "yes" and "no"
- b. Functional muscular stimulation using electrodes to stimulate the muscles of speech
- c. A laptop computer driven by the patient's eye movements
- d. A spelling board

202. In treating status epilepticus, the FIRST drug to administer intravenously is:
- a. Fosphenytoin
- b. Diazepam
- c. Lorazepam
- d. Phenobarbital

203. Patients with idiopathic intracranial hypertension should be followed:
- a. Slit lamp examination
- b. Quantitative visual field examination
- c. Visual acuity determination
- d. Retinal angiography

204. When a patient with narcolepsy experiences an episode of excessive:
- a. He cannot be aroused until the episode passes
- b. He usually awakens feeling refreshed, although not necessarily for long
- c. He has sufficient warning to make himself safe before falling asleep
- d. He does not dream

205. Careful temperature monitoring of patients following acute stroke is essential primarily because:
- a. Hyperthermia predisposes the patient to nonneurologic complications such as myocardial infarction and cardiac arrhythmia
- b. Hyperthermia destabilizes autoregulation of cerebral blood flow
- c. Hyperthermia increases the risk of infarct extension
- d. Hyperthermia contributes to increased intracranial pressure

206. Following recombinant tissue plasminogen activator (rt-PA) for acute ischemic stroke, the patient:
- a. Moves to ICU on a heparin infusion
- b. Moves to ICU and begins oral warfarin
- c. Moves to ICU and begins anti-platelet therapy
- d. Moves to ICU with bleeding precautions

207. Families of individuals with Alzheimer's disease should be educated that Alzheimer's disease is:
    a. A terminal disease
    b. An acute syndrome
    c. A subacute syndrome
    d. A reversible dementia

208. Patients with amyotrophic lateral sclerosis experience extended survival time and time to requiring tracheostomy when they are treated with:
    a. High-dose vitamin E
    b. High dose vitamin D
    c. Riluzole
    d. Creatine 5-10 g/d

209. A step-wise decline in cognitive function is MOST characteristic of:
    a. Alzheimer's disease
    b. Normal pressure hydrocephalus
    c. Dementia caused by depression
    d. Multi-infarct dementia

210. The factor which constitutes the GREATEST risk for multi-infarct dementia is:
    a. Cigarette smoking
    b. Hypertension
    c. Diabetes
    d. Elevated cholesterol

211. The MOST essential element in treating obstructive sleep apnea is:
    a. Continuous positive airway pressure (CPAP)
    b. Weight loss
    c. Surgery to widen the pharynx
    d. Lifestyle adjustments, including sleep hygiene and avoidance of cigarettes and alcohol

212. A patient presents with agitation progressing toward delirium and is discovered to have elevated serum ammonia and transaminases. His agitation is attributed to hepatic encephalopathy, and a work-up is undertaken to establish the cause of his liver failure. While the work-up is in progress, appropriate treatment includes:
    a. Lactulose
    b. Benzodiazepine medication
    c. Antipsychotic medication
    d. Anticonvulsant medication

213. An elderly woman with early stage Alzheimer's disease enters the hospital for treatment of congestive heart failure in her usual mental state. After two days, she is hemodynamically more stable, but she develops fluctuating inattention and disorientation with periods of agitation and yelling. While a medical work-up is in progress, the bes approach to her care is to:
    a. Move her to ICU for closer monitoring
    b. Keep the patient's room darkened and quiet
    c. Limit visitors to five minute intervals
    d. Establish a normal diurnal rhythm of activity and rest

214. The most sensitive laboratory marker for neuromyelitis optica is:
    a. Oligoclonal bands in the cerebrospinal fluid
    b. Elevated IgG synthesis as calculated from serum and CSF measurements
    c. Serum NMO IgG antibody
    d. Serum anti-Purkinje cell antibodies

215. A patient presenting with a rapidly progressive course consisting of fever, focal abnormalities on neurologic examination, and evidence of increased intracranial pressure is MOST likely to have:
    a. Brain abscess
    b. Viral meningitis
    c. Intracranial hemorrhage
    d. Metabolic encephalopathy

216. Craniopharyngiomas are generally:
    a. Solid rather than cystic
    b. Suprasellar in location, with neurologic symptoms similar to those of pituitary adenoma
    c. Histologically malignant, but actually unlikely to recur
    d. Responsive to chemotherapy

217. Post-polio syndrome:
    a. Is more likely to occur in patients who made a poor recovery from the initial illness than in patients who made a good recovery
    b. Is associated with elevated IgG synthesis rate
    c. Can cause sleep apnea
    d. Is associated with decreased amplitude and duration of motor action potentials on electromyography (EMG)

218. A patient who presents with pure mental neuropathy (numb chin syndrome) is MOST likely to have:
    a. Multiple sclerosis
    b. Trigeminal neuralgia
    c. Mononeuritis multiplex
    d. Metastatic cancer

219. A patient who has sustained closed head trauma is treated with a hypothermia protocol for rapidly increasing intracranial pressure. During hypothermia and during rewarming, the laboratory parameter it is MOST important to follow is:
    a. Serum sodium
    b. Serum potassium
    c. Serum calcium
    d. Urine osmolality

220. A young patient presenting with Bell's palsy should always be evaluated for:
    a. Multiple sclerosis
    b. Stroke
    c. Metastatic malignancy
    d. Diabetes mellitus

Answers and Explanations

1. C: Treatment for bacterial meningitis is urgent; the risk of mortality is too great to wait for a definitive bacteriologic diagnosis. Drug selection targets the organisms most likely to be present on clinical grounds and on the known antibiotic sensitivities of those organisms in the region and in the specific institution. These sensitivities vary geographically and evolve over time. Because of the seriousness of the infection, bactericidal antibiotics are preferable. If dexamethasone is included in the treatment regimen, it should be started before – or at least concomitant with – the first dose of antibiotic as the first phase of bacterial death can intensify the inflammatory response.

2. D: Unlike bacterial meningitis, viral meningitis cannot be transmitted from person to person via direct contact or airborne secretions. The viruses that cause aseptic meningitis in humans are called arboviruses and are transmitted by mosquitoes. Some of these viruses also cause encephalitis. Serial neurologic examination is important to detect focal neurologic abnormalities as soon as they develop, since viral meningitis is often accompanied by encephalitis. Some focal deficits can be life threatening, such as dysphagia. Any deterioration in level of consciousness should also be noted as promptly as possible so that the cause can be addressed, for example, by reversing increased intracranial pressure. Deteriorating level of consciousness is a poor prognostic sign. Hyperthermia in any setting can result in permanent brain damage.

3. A: The most important nursing precaution to take prior to lumbar puncture is to look for any evidence of a clotting disorder, because bleeding into the limited spinal subarachnoid space can produce a hematoma that entraps or compresses the cauda equina. The physician will already have assessed the risk of herniation due to increased intracranial pressure with or without a space-occupying lesion. It is advisable to have the patient attend to bathroom needs prior to the lumbar puncture so that he doesn't have to sit or stand following the procedure, but this is a lower priority than checking the coagulation studies. No restriction of food or liquid is necessary prior to lumbar puncture. Patient education is a part of preparation for any procedure, but again, the most pressing nursing intervention is to review the coagulation studies.

4. A: Lyme disease is caused by the spirochete B. burgdorferi, which is not quickly killed by antibiotics. If the diagnosis is made before neurologic, cardiac, or joint involvement, then antibiotic treatment can usually be completed orally at home. The patient needs to understand that treatment is not complete until the last prescribed dose has been taken. IV antibiotics may be required if the disease has progressed to involve the CNS, heart, or joints. In that case, the patient will remain in hospital or be discharged home with home nursing support. In either case, completing the entire course of treatment is essential. The patient should understand that especially if treatment has been started early in the course of the disease, he is very likely NOT immune to subsequent infection with B. burgdorferi, because his immune system may not have had sufficient time to mount an effective response. The patient should understand precautions against repeat infection. The infective agent is tick-borne, so the patient should avoid wooded environments and use insect repellents and wear protective clothing whenever he cannot avoid tick habitats. He should inspect himself and his pets regularly for ticks and understand the correct and incorrect methods for removing any ticks he may find. B. burgdorferi is not transmitted from human to human, so isolation is not required at any stage. The patient should be aware that Lyme disease is a chronic

illness, and many individuals experience intermittent long-term symptoms such as arthralgias, headache and lethargy, but actual permanent joint damage is, in fact, unlikely.

5. C: The goal of disease-modifying treatment for multiple sclerosis is not cure or reversal of existing symptoms. Rather, the goal is to reduce the frequency and severity of exacerbations and to delay development of disability. For this reason, patients are easily frustrated even by successful therapy, because they cannot see concrete, positive improvement. Patients and their families often benefit by repeated reminders about the actual goals of treatment, even if they are not expressing frustration. Since depression can be a primary symptom of MS, a reaction to a particular loss associated with the disease, or a side effect of interferon treatment, the treatment team should always be alert to possible depression, but the first-line intervention in this case is education. If the patient is doing well neurologically and not experiencing unmanageable side effects, it is not appropriate to propose changing drugs.

6. B:Given her symptoms and signs, this patient likely has meningitis. She will certainly need IV antibiotics as soon as possible. Given her age and close living quarters, meningococcal meningitis (caused by Neisseria meningitidis) is the likely pathogen; her rapid course and the presence of petechiae suggest she is at risk for a fulminant presentation, which can include circulatory collapse. IV access may be needed not only for antibiotics, but also for fluids and pressors. Although she may ultimately require intubation, the IV is urgent immediately. Meningococcal meningitis is largely preventable by immunization, but immunization will not prevent disease in persons who have already been exposed. Close contacts should receive chemoprophylaxis with antibiotics. Vaccination is still appropriate for others in the environment beyond the immediate contacts, as vaccination may prevent a secondary outbreak.

7. B: Exercise is at least as important for individuals with multiple sclerosis as for others to maintain cardiovascular health, skeletal integrity, and bone strength and exercise confers psychological benefits as well. Because elevated core temperature can temporarily worsen MS symptoms, some people with MS are reluctant to exercise. The fastest way to lower core body temperature is by ingesting cool liquids. External cooling, as with vests, is costly and cumbersome. Dressing lightly throughout exercise is sensible, but to actually reduce core temperature, drinking cool liquids is the most effective approach.

8. A: In any patient whose myasthenia gravis is rapidly deteriorating, the most life-threatening development is respiratory failure. This is restrictive rather than obstructive respiratory failure, based on inability of the muscles of respiration to contract sufficiently to move air into the chest. Unlike obstructive failure, restrictive failure is not accompanied by overt respiratory symptoms, such as wheezing or gasping, and the patient may not be particularly hypoxic or even feel short of breath until complete respiratory failure is imminent. For this reason, the physical examination and arterial blood gases are inadequate measures of pulmonary function, and regular measurement of vital capacity is mandatory. The physician should determine in advance a value at which semi-elective intubation will be instituted in order to avoid a respiratory emergency. It is also important to evaluate other muscle groups, particularly the muscles of swallowing, as aspiration of secretions is also a very serious event. All patients should be carefully monitored for possible adverse events when they start a new medication. A wide range of drugs can worsen myasthenia, and while these

are to be avoided, they may sometimes be watchfully given when the potential benefit is judged to outweigh the risk.

9. D: For myasthenic patients with difficulty swallowing, a liquid diet poses more risk of aspiration than does a mechanical soft diet. The mechanical soft diet includes foods that are easily chewed, such as scrambled eggs, pasta, and cooked vegetables. Foods to avoid include tough meats, nuts, crusty breads, and raw fruits. While anticholinergic medications should be timed for maximum effectiveness during essential activities such as eating, the use of sustained-release medications makes it unnecessary to medicate before every meal or snack. Small meals make fatigue of the muscles of mastication less likely. It is best not to eat when at risk for aspiration, but it is usually not necessary to go hungry in the face of mild fatigue. Patients should be encouraged to know and honor their own body's signals.

10. D: The key issue is that once a patient loses the ability to swallow or breathe because of ALS, that ability will not return, and intervention is not temporary. Some ALS patients will want to take advantage of every life-saving measure and some will reject prolonged ventilatory support at the end of life. Many will be ambivalent and need consultation with
family members, ethicists, clergy, or other advisors. There may be disagreement among family members. The discussion should be initiated early, respectfully, and supportively.

11. D: Respiratory failure is a common feature of Guillain-Barré syndrome and occurs because of neuromuscular weakness, not intrinsic lung pathology. When the cause of respiratory failure is neuromuscular, the patient may deteriorate very abruptly without having had symptoms or signs of hypoxia in advance. Relying on the clinical picture alone or
supplemented by pulse oximetry or even arterial blood gases can be falsely reassuring. Once the vital capacity falls below 12-15 mL/kg, the patient is at risk for ventilatory failure, and intubation should proceed regardless of the patient's comfort level or other signs. Of course, measuring the respiratory rate and regularly auscultating the lungs are also important measures, but the most important element of respiratory monitoring is frequent vital capacity determination.

12. C: Patients with Guillain-Barré syndrome are at risk for deep vein thrombosis (DVT) because of prolonged immobility or reduced mobility. Compression boots can injure peripheral nerves already compromised by autoimmune inflammatory demyelination, so
compression is not a good choice for these patients. Peroneal nerve palsy is a particular risk. Minidoses of heparin are sufficient to prevent DVT. This approach carries fewer risks, is more immediately effective, and is more rapidly reversible than oral warfarin. Aspirin is not effective DVT prophylaxis, irreversibly damages platelets, and carries a risk of gastritis,
especially in a critically ill patient. Because of the risk of peripheral nerve injury, positioning and turning are especially important considerations in the care of these immobilized patients.

13. A: Total opioid requirement is minimized with sustained-release medication taken time-contingently. The patient will likely have a prescription for a few tablets of an immediate-release medication for break-through pain. Tolerance to adverse side effects of the opioids, including respiratory suppression, develops very rapidly. If the patient has received opioid medication in the hospital before discharge, tolerance to respiratory suppression has already

developed. The patient should, however, have pro-active bowel management while on opioids to prevent constipation, especially if there has been autonomic nervous system involvement.

In educating the patient and family about addiction, it is important to explain to them that tolerance (needing more medication to get the same level of pain relief) and dependence (experiencing unpleasant symptoms with abrupt withdrawal) are purely physiologic responses and can be managed in cooperation with the physician. Addiction is a completely different phenomenon from tolerance and dependence and is unlikely in the absence of pre-existing risk factors for addiction. While neuropathic pain often responds to a variety of non-opioid drugs, including anticonvulsants and tricyclic antidepressants, the pain of Guillain-Barré syndrome is often so severe as to require opioids.

14. B: The eye on the affected side in Bell's palsy does not close completely, so the eye has to be protected. Patches provide mechanical protection against foreign debris lodging in the eye and may be indicated in windy conditions or sometimes for sleep. The most important on- going consideration, however, is maintaining lubrication of the eye. The cornea is easily injured if it is not kept moist, and the eye may be dry, not only because of incomplete closure, but also because of reduced or absent tear production due to the cranial nerve VII dysfunction. Lubrication with tears and ointments is vital. Various devices such as eyelid weights can promote eye closure, but the first line of protection is lubrication. Facial exercises and nerve stimulation may be helpful in promoting recovery, but they will not protect the eye in the short term.

15. B: Most patients with multiple sclerosis do not have bladder symptoms at the time of diagnosis, but the majority of patients with MS will have bladder dysfunction of some kind at some point in their disease course. Bladder dysfunction in MS is often asymptomatic and usually consists of both detrusor hyperreflexia and incomplete emptying. This combination is known as detrusor external sphincter dyssynergia (DESD.) The patient may experience repeated bladder hyperdistention without any awareness of the problem, and this can lead, over time, to irreversible bladder flaccidity and incontinence and predisposes the patient to infection as well. Frequent timed voiding is a simple preventive measure that all patients with MS should learn and practice. Some neurologists feel that a urologist should be made a part of the patient's treatment team before there is any bladder disturbance, but this is optional. Self-catheterization is an easy skill to master and need not be taught unless there is an actual need for it.

16. A: Humans are the definitive hosts for T. solium. Infection can be passed from human to human via fecal contamination without an intermediate host, and infection can be acquired by ingesting undercooked pork that contains parasites. Good handwashing practice is the first line of defense against spread of cysticercosis. Proper precautions in handling and cooking pork are also important, and travelers from the United States should drink only bottled or boiled water when in endemic countries. There is no vaccine against T. solium. Immunoserologic assays may be positive in individuals who do not have active clinical disease and are not actively shedding parasites. Antihelminthic treatment is not indicated in every patient with neurocysticercosis and is, in fact, contraindicated in some because of the risk of hydrocephalus if inflammation around degenerating cysticerci obstructs ventricular outflow.

17. A: Creutzfeldt-Jakob disease is caused by prions, abnormally folded proteins, which can be acquired by contact with contaminated tissues (e.g. cornea transplants or dural grafts before the mid-1980s) or biological products (e.g. human cadaver-derived growth hormone before 1985.) An estimated 5-15% of cases are considered to be genetic in which case, a gene that causes abnormal folding of a protein is inherited; most cases are sporadic. Universal precautions apply, and certain instruments that come in contact with the patient's bodily fluids should not be reused, but isolation precautions are not required because ordinary human-to human transmission does not occur. Symptoms vary according to the parts of the central nervous system involved, and psychiatric manifestations often dominate early in the course. The disease follows an inexorable course of progressive dementia and is fatal within 13 months. Total care is required during the final months of life. The patient and
family need support to address end-of-life issues as effectively as possible.

18. D: The pathophysiology of AIDS dementia complex is complex and includes entry of HIV into the brain within infected monocytes, widespread neuronal damage by cellular proteins and verotoxins, abnormal patterns of neurotransmitter release, and increased free intraneuronal calcium. HAART is thought to reduce entry of HIV into the central nervous system and to reduce neuronal damage by HIV once it has entered the CNS. HAART has significantly reduced the incidence of ADC in HIV-positive patients. In addition, HAART reduces severity and prolongs survival in cases of established ADC. Some patients with ADC also experience cognitive improvement with HAART treatment. There are no data to support the use of cholinesterase inhibitors.

19. B: Fatigue is a nearly universal complaint in multiple sclerosis. Primary MS fatigue is fatigue attributable directly to the disease process of the MS itself; secondary MS fatigue is fatigue due to other MS symptoms, such as urinary frequency that interferes with sleep or motor weakness that adds an energy toll to ordinary activities. Medications to manage symptoms of multiple sclerosis or other conditions can induce daytime drowsiness or contribute to daytime sleepiness by interfering with sleep at night. In addition, MS patients who report fatigue should be evaluated for causes of fatigue unrelated to their MS diagnosis, such as hypothyroidism, anemia, or sleep apnea, just like any other patient.

Many medications are tried empirically to treat primary MS fatigue, but only modafinil has been shown to be effective when compared with placebo and evaluated on the Fatigue Severity Scale. Pharmacologic management can be helpful, but in the absence of a patient-directed regimen of activity pacing, medications alone are of limited value. It is often difficult for patients to pace activities time-contingently and manage their energy pro-actively, and it is appropriate for the nurse to remind patients and their families of this strategy frequently. Many patients tend to overexert themselves on days when they feel energetic and then take the next day or days to rest and recover. Activity pacing allows the patient to conserve energy and avoid compensatory down time. Occupational therapy can also be helpful, particularly for patients with significant motor impairments who benefit from finding more ergonomically effective ways of accomplishing routine tasks.

20. C: Neutral position is ideal because allowing the head to turn to either side can cause jugular vein compression, which could contribute to increased intracranial pressure. Flexion causes

traction on the meninges and can be painful; this is the basis of the Kernig's sign. Extension can also be uncomfortable. There is no advantage to fetal position, except
during lumbar puncture.

21. B: Comment: In addition to monitoring the PTT to ensure adequate anticoagulation without undue risk of bleeding, it is essential to monitor the platelet count daily to look for early evidence of heparin-induced thrombocytopenia (HIT.) This is an immune reaction induced by heparin. Clinical manifestations range from innocuous petechiae on the skin to
thrombotic and thromboembolic complications of the skin, extremities and internal organ systems. The reaction is potentially fatal. The earliest sign of HIT is an otherwise unexplained drop in the platelet count. HIT can also occur on a delayed basis, with onset a week or more after heparin treatment has been discontinued. Generalized hypersensitivity reactions may also occur, manifesting as urticaria, rhinitis, or asthma. The PT is useful in assessing adequacy of anticoagulation with warfarin.

22. A: Once the patient has had bleeding from an intracranial aneurysm, there remains a risk of rebleeding. The incidence of rebleeding following the initial presentation may be as high as 30%. Straining at stool raises intracranial pressure and poses a particular risk for rebleeding. The aneurysm patient is placed at bedrest and often has severe head pain requiring opioid medication, with the attendant side effect of reduced intestinal peristalsis. These factors combined predictably lead to constipation, so a good bowel regimen has to be
instituted proactively. It is important to prevent straining at stool, because this increases intracranial pressure. Waiting for constipation to develop is waiting too long, because it is more difficult to treat established constipation than to just prevent it, and because by the time the patient becomes constipated, he will have entered the time of greatest risk for rebleeding.

Seizure precautions are important for the patient's safety, but seizure precautions only keep the patient safe in the event of seizures; only anticonvulsant medication can actually prevent seizures. Measures to prevent deep vein thrombophlebitis are important, but they do not protect the patient against aneurysmal bleeding.

At one time, it was common practice to limit fluid intake in patients with SAH as part of an over-all strategy of keeping blood pressure low. In fact, however, volume restriction and excessively low blood pressure both increase the risk of vasospasm and rebleeding.

23. D: Blood pressure is often elevated immediately following SAH, as a response to increased intracranial pressure. Blood pressure management should aim to keep the systolic pressure between 120 and 150 mm Hg without excessive vasodilatation, which can promote rupture of an untreated aneurysm. The pressure should be high enough to prevent rebleeding due to vasospasm and low enough to rebleeding due to hypertension.

24. C: Although antidiuretic hormone (ADH) may be elevated in the immediate aftermath of subarachnoid hemorrhage (SAH), ADH levels decline spontaneously in the ensuing days, and urine and serum electrolytes are consistent with primary sodium wasting, not syndrome of inappropriate ADH (SIADH.) Although sodium restriction is appropriate for treatment of ADH, it is inappropriate

- 133 -

for treating primary sodium wasting, which requires sodium replacement. In addition, the SAH patient requires volume expansion to avoid cerebral vasospasm and the attendant risk of rebleeding.

25. A: Regardless of treatment for intracranial aneurysm, outcomes do not vary by age. Costs do increase in proportion to age and length of hospital stay. Early surgical repair can improve outcome and shorten hospital stay. Outcome data is a relevant and admissible factor in guiding treatment choices, but age is not a relevant or ethical criterion on which to base treatment choices for intracranial aneurysm.

26. D: Thrombolysis with recombinant intravenous tissue-type plasminogen activator (rt-PA) can restore perfusion to ischemic brain tissue. Early in the course of ischemic stroke, necrosis of ischemic tissue can be prevented with thrombolysis.

After three hours, the likelihood of saving the ischemic tissue declines and the risk of hemorrhagic transformation of the ischemic infarct increases. Studies have established 3 hours as the longest duration of symptoms within which risk outweighs benefit for rt-PA. Studies have shown that outcome is not related to age or sex. Thrombolysis cannot be attempted in an anticoagulated patient. If the patient has been on heparin, he cannot undergo thrombolysis until the PTT is normal. If the patient has been on warfarin, the patient cannot undergo thrombolysis until the INR is > 1.7. Anticoagulants and anti-platelet drugs should not be given for the first 24 hours following rt-PA.

Serum glucose should be no less than 50 mg/dl. In the hours and days following thrombolysis, serum glucose should be managed to avoid hyperglycemia as well as hypoglycemia, as hyperglycemia can predispose to both hemorrhage and hypoperfusion.

27. C: Blood pressure monitoring and stabilization is critically important in the hours following carotid endarterectomy in order to avoid both hyperperfusion and hypoperfusion syndromes. Following carotid endarterectomy, abrupt restoration of arterial perfusion can lead to intracerebral hemorrhage. This is a particular risk until cerebral blood flow autoregulation normalizes. In addition to disrupted cerebral blood flow autoregulation, there is also disruption of the normal systemic baroreceptor responses in patients immediately following surgical manipulation of the carotid artery, so systemic blood pressure may be difficult to regulate just when the brain is most vulnerable to alterations in flow. In this setting, hypertension poses a risk of hemorrhage, and hypotension poses a risk of cerebral ischemia. Blood pressure should be monitored continuously, and overcorrection is to be avoided. For most patients, a systolic pressure between 120 and 130 mm Hg is optimal.

28. C: Especially with injury to the frontal and temporal lobes, stroke patients may lack self-monitoring and display socially inappropriate behaviors such as disregarding personal hygiene or making socially unacceptable sexual advances. Although these behaviors are involuntary and should not be judged, neither should they be ignored. It is important to make the patient aware of unacceptable behavior and reassure the patient and family that this behavior is a result of organic brain injury, is not a reflection upon the patient's character, and can be brought under control in time. It is helpful to state and repeat expectations clearly and to maintain a predictable routine help

to minimize unwanted behaviors. Psychiatric care, including psychoactive medications, may be needed, but with or without psychiatric input, the patient and family absolutely need both explanation and reassurance about the origin of distressing behaviors.

29. B: Interference with vitamin K and the synthesis of clotting factors that depend upon vitamin K is the mechanism by which warfarin maintains anticoagulation. Taking vitamin K undermines anticoagulation with warfarin. Leafy green vegetables contain vitamin K. Patients should not avoid this class of foods, because they also provide fiber, folic acid, antioxidants, trace minerals, and other nutrients. While taking warfarin, however, they should keep their intake of leafy green vegetables as consistent as possible, avoiding unaccustomed excesses or unaccustomed abstinence from these foods. Plant-derived nutritional supplements should also be avoided. Patients should avoid cranberries and cranberry juice because they can augment the effects of warfarin as can ginseng, gingko, and certain botanicals such as St. John's wort. Alcohol is to be avoided altogether because of its inhibitory effect on the liver enzymes that break down warfarin. The therapeutic range for warfarin is narrow, and any factor that influences its actions or metabolism should be either strictly controlled or avoided altogether. The patient should not add or discontinue any prescription or over-the counter medication while on warfarin without consulting the physician who is prescribing and monitoring the warfarin. With proper management of the medication, occult GI bleeding is not to be anticipated, and iron supplementation is not required.

30. C: CT scan is often normal early in the course of herpes simplex encephalitis. MRI is more frequently abnormal, but the characteristic frontotemporal areas of hemorrhage are non-specific. A 4-fold rise in serum antibody titer is reliable but does not ensue until the convalescent stage – if the patient survives. The EEG changes are also non-specific. The only early laboratory indicator of herpes simplex encephalitis is the presence of viral DNA in the CSF. If this testing is not available, then the decision to treat must be made on clinical grounds supplemented by whatever imaging and laboratory data are available. Symptoms can be rapidly progressive, and if treatment is delayed until the onset of coma, mortality is over 30%.

31. A: Although anticoagulation with heparin is standard treatment in the acute phase of management of the patient with cerebral venous thrombosis, the risk of converting an ischemic infarct to a hemorrhagic infarct is substantial; as many as 40% of CVT patients actually have hemorrhagic infarcts even before starting IV heparin. Acute changes in neurologic status of patients with CVT should be treated as if for intracerebral hemorrhage pending further evaluation.

32. D: Patients with acute hemorrhagic cerebral infarction are at greatest risk for increased intracranial pressure and its attendant complications, including transtentorial herniation. Not only do these patients need extremely close monitoring, but if increased intracranial pressure is not responsive to simple measures such as positioning and mannitol, then more invasive measures may be needed rapidly. These measures may include ventriculostomy and hyperventilation. Patients with hemorrhagic cerebral infraction are also at greater risk than patients in the other three categories for accelerated systemic hypertension.

33. B: The risk of bleeding from an arteriovenous malformation is probably slightly increased during pregnancy. Theoretically, the temporary increases in intracranial pressure associated with the transition stage of labor could contribute to bleeding from an AVM, but vaginal delivery is not absolutely contraindicated for a woman with an AVM.

None of the disease-modifying agents for MS is approved for use during pregnancy. When pregnancy can be planned, a patient should discontinue disease-modifying therapy several months before attempting to become pregnant. Pregnancy usually has a good effect on MS, and the incidence of exacerbations during pregnancy is lower than at any other time in the reproductive cycle. The post-partum period, however, is a time of increased incidence of exacerbations, and many neurologists advise patients to forgo breastfeeding in order to resume disease modifying therapy immediately after delivery.

Pregnancy itself does not have a predictable effect on the course of myasthenia. About a third of women feel better symptomatically while pregnant while another third feel worse, and the remainder feel no different. Data concerning safety of anticholinergic medications during pregnancy are inconclusive regarding possible harm to the fetus. Most women who have been requiring anticholinergic medication prior to pregnancy will continue to need it while pregnant.

34. D: Although the annual risk of bleeding from an unruptured intracerebral AVM is low, the percentage cumulative lifetime risk can be estimated at 105 minus the patient's age in years at presentation. This risk is higher for aneurysms that have already bled once. Other factors also increase the risk of bleeding. Smaller AVMs have a higher risk, presumably because of higher pressures within the feeding artery. Hemorrhage risk is also greater for lesions that have only a single draining vein. Larger AVMs are less likely to bleed but are more likely to cause seizures, either because they are more likely to exert a mass effect on adjacent cerebral cortex or because of relative ischemia induced by shunting of larger volumes of blood away from parts of the cortex. Average mortality with the initial bleed from an AVM is between 6% and 30% and each hemorrhage increases the risk of subsequent hemorrhage.

35. A: Until autoregulation of cerebral blood flow is re-established, the risk of bleeding is significant. The patients who are at risk of vasospasm are those who have had subarachnoid hemorrhage (SAH) due to a ruptured intracranial aneurysm, but vasospasm is not the main concern in the postoperative AVM patient. Cerebral venous hypertension is a concern preoperatively in patients who have high-flow AVMs, but it is not a major postoperative concern. SIADH is not a common complication in postsurgical AVM patients, and the patient should be kept well hydrated.

36. B: The single greatest risk factor for lacunar strokes is hypertension. To the extent that thrombosis is part of the pathophysiology of lacunar infarcts, it is secondary to microatheroma of small penetrating arteries, a condition promoted by sustained systemic arterial hypertension. Cigarette smoking and diabetes mellitus are lesser risk factors for lacunar infarction. Anticoagulation may be considered only in the minority of cases in which a cardiac embolic source appears to be the cause of lacunar infarcts.

37. C: Although this patient did not experience blunt trauma, he has likely had non-traumatic neck injury. His unilateral pain accompanied by ipsilateral monocular blindness suggests a right internal carotid arterial dissection with embolization to the right ophthalmic artery. A partial Horner's syndrome is a very common manifestation of carotid dissection because of the location of the sympathetic fibers to the face. The syndrome is partial - no anhydrosis – because the sympathetic fibers to the facial sweat glands are adjacent to the external carotid artery. Carotid dissection can be caused by surprisingly mild external force as well as by major blunt trauma. Mild injuries that can result in carotid dissection include whiplash, coughing, sneezing, and sexual activity. Some dissections occur spontaneously in the setting of fibromuscular Dysplasia or connective tissue disorders such as Ehlers-Danlos syndrome. Incidence is highest in young adults. Cerebral ischemia in the form of stroke or TIA occurs in at least 75% of patients with carotid dissection. A carotid bruit, if present, may aid in diagnosis, but in the majority of cases, there is no bruit.

38. A: Hemifacial spasm is a syndrome, not a diagnosis. Hemifacial spasm is often caused by an aberrant blood vessel irritating the facial nerve at the cerebellopontine angle. Other compressive lesions may also produce hemifacial spasm. In this case, there was no aberrant vessel and presumably no other compressive lesion. The patient is atypical because of her age as hemifacial spasm presents most often in the 5th or 6th decade of life. Although hemifacial spasm can occur on an idiopathic basis, underlying neurologic disease has to be considered, especially given the patient's age. She should be re-evaluated for multiple sclerosis, especially since this diagnosis could impact her decisions concerning if, when, and how to have children. Botulinum toxin may relieve her symptoms regardless of the cause, but further investigation at this point is essential. Some patients with orofacial dyskinesia have underlying dental abnormalities (often edentulousness) but the condition should be clinically distinguishable from hemifacial spasm and rarely affects young people, so dental consultation is not likely to produce useful information in this case. Psychiatric consultation may help the patient to cope with cosmetically distressing problem, but it will not yield diagnostic information or alleviate her symptoms.

39. C: Hyperventilation is a strategy for short-term management of increased intracranial pressure (ICP.) The resulting hypocapnia causes vasoconstriction. This is intended to reduce both cerebral blood flow and ICP, but sometimes only cerebral blood flow is actually decreased, and the effect may be inconsistent in different areas of the brain. Even when successful, the benefit is only temporary. For these reasons, hyperventilation is a less than ideal approach and should only be used as a temporizing measure until a more definitive approach such as ventriculostomy can be instituted. Furthermore, rebound ICP often ensues if hyperventilation is discontinued abruptly.

40. A: Hemineglect syndrome is usually refractory to treatment. The patient may never fully recognize the affected side of his body as truly belonging to him. He, his family, the hospital staff, and ultimately his associates outside the hospital will need to make accommodations to cope with this deficit. It will be important to assist the patient with bathing and grooming of the unrecognized body parts and to help him avoid injury. Emotionally, the deficit may be more distressing to family members than to the patient, and they will need support in finding coping strategies. Techniques of behavioral modification, electrical or magnetic stimulation of the body parts or cerebral hemisphere are generally not successful.

41. C: In laboratory models, it is more difficult to induce experimental autoimmune encephalitis (EAE) in animals that have been pre-treated with Vitamin D. In animals with established EAE, those treated with Vitamin D have a milder course. In a 20-year epidemiologic study of 187,563 nurses, a negative correlation was demonstrated between Vitamin D intake and incidence of MS. Offspring of a parent with MS have a risk of developing MS between 1 in 100 and 1 in 40, compared with the average risk of 1 in 750 for the general population. MS is thought to develop through interaction of a variety of environmental factors on a polygenic hereditary substrate. Clinical trials of Vitamin D in humans with MS are now in progress. Vitamin D deficiency has been implicated as a causative factor in numerous autoimmune diseases and malignancies, including multiple sclerosis, rheumatoid arthritis, diabetes, and cancers of the prostate, colon, ovary, and breast. Daily vitamin D requirement and normal serum Vitamin D levels have been underestimated, and these parameters are being revised upward.

42. C: ROM exercises should begin as soon as possible to promote motor recovery and prevent contractures. Only fractures or other medical contraindications should be allowed to delay ROM exercises. If the patient is not fully conscious, passive ROM can still be initiated, progressing to active assisted and then active ROM as the patient recovers. Spasticity (hyperactive deep tendon reflexes and exaggerated motor response to altered joint position) and synergy (simultaneous contraction of multiple muscle groups in response to displacement at a single joint) are stages of motor recovery following stroke. ROM should be started even before these stages during the initial phase of flaccidity whenever possible.

43. A: The fundamental premise of the Bobath approach is that the sensation of movement is learned, and sensory learning precedes motor learning. The patient is assisted to re-establish basic patterns of posture, truncal support, and equilibrium, and through the sensory experience of these healthy patterns, the patient can re-establish normal movements within the limits imposed by the residual neurologic deficits.

44. B: Placing the patient's unaffected side closest to the bed allows him to place his weight preferentially on the stronger leg. While there is an imperative to encourage the patient to use the affected side as much as possible, it is not acceptable to compromise safety to do so. Angling the chair allows the chair to be place as close as possible to the bed.

45. D: Supervised feeding can begin when it has been demonstrated that the patient has normal bilateral gag reflex and normal swallow reflex, both of which can be determined by simple bedside examination. A barium swallow with videofluoroscopy is not necessary if these tests are normal. Depending on the type of difficulty a patient has, different textures of food may be best; in some cases, solids are easier and safer than liquids. If the muscles of mastication are weak on one side, the patient should place food on the unaffected side, at least when first resuming an oral diet.

46. A: Blood in the brain parenchyma is obvious on non-contrast CT scan. CT is more efficient than MRI in this setting. Lumbar puncture is the most sensitive way to detect blood in the cerebrospinal fluid, and lumbar puncture is the definitive procedure to diagnose subarachnoid hemorrhage. Blood in the subarachnoid space is usually not obvious on imaging studies unless the hemorrhage has been massive.

47. D: Labetalol is usually the drug of choice for control of hypertension in the setting of acute stroke because it is short-acting, easily titrated, and does not cause cerebral vasodilation. Nitroprusside and nimodipine both cause cerebral vasodilation, which is undesirable following stroke. Nimodipine is used in the setting of subarachnoid hemorrhage from intracranial aneurysm, because it reduces cerebral vasospasm, which is a risk factor for rebleeding. Furosemide is undesirable not only because of vasodilation, but also because of its diuretic effect. In general, unless the systolic pressure exceeds 220 mm Hg or the diastolic pressure exceeds 120 mm Hg, antihypertensive drugs are avoided early in the course of stroke in order to avoid hypoperfusion. It is important to avoid lowering the blood pressure too rapidly.

48. B: Hematogenous spread is the most common means of entry of an infective agent into the central nervous system. Organisms that are well tolerated in certain tissue compartments, such as the pharynx, become deadly when they reach the meninges via hematogenous spread. Entry via skull injury is less common both because penetrating injuries to the skull are relatively infrequent and because prophylactic antibiotic treatment is usually a part of the medical management of such injuries. The slow virus of Creutzfeldt-Jakob disease may enter the CNS via contaminated surgical instruments or contaminated transplanted tissues. Some organisms, such as the rabies virus, can reach the CNS via peripheral nerves. Herpes simplex may reach the CNS either hematogenously or via the peripheral nerves. Infection can rarely reach the CNS via congenital dural defects or occult encephaloceles.

49. D: N. meningitidis (meningococcus) is the leading cause of bacterial meningitis in adolescents and young adults. In half of patients, presentation includes a petechial rash, purpura, or ecchymosis, which can aid in diagnosis. Petechiae may involve the conjunctivae and mucous membranes as well as the skin. In about 10% of cases, the presentation is fulminant with septicemia, circulatory collapse (Waterhouse-Friderichsen syndrome), and disseminated intravascular coagulation (DIC.) Untreated, these fulminant cases can be fatal within hours. Preferred antibiotic treatment for meningococcal meningitis is with a third-generation cephalosporin. Fulminating meningococcemia, even without meningeal involvement, also requires blood pressure support and prompt treatment with adrenal corticosteroids.

50. C: Hematogenous spread from distant sites is the most common source of infection leading to brain abscess. In addition to the lung and heart, the skin can also be a source of infection. Although the antibiotic era brought about a drastic reduction in the incidence of brain abscess attributable to direct spread of infection from adjacent sites such as the middle ear and mastoid, otitis media and mastoiditis still account together for approximately 40% of brain abscesses, and sinuitis accounts for nearly another 10%, so investigation of recent head and neck infections – especially if only partially treated – remains an important part of the nursing assessment of a patient when brain abscess is suspected or diagnosed.

51. C: While the overall prevalence of cerebral aneurysms is greater than the prevalence of AVMs, the likelihood of rupture of an AVM is greater than the likelihood of rupture of an intracranial aneurysm of any size. Because carotid cavernous fistulas usually make themselves known by symptoms related to their mass effect (pulsatile tinnitus, diplopia, exophthalmos, and headache,) intervention is possible before a hemorrhagic event.

52. B: Non-contrast CT of the brain is the most sensitive test for recent subarachnoid hemorrhage with a sensitivity rate of 98% in the first 12 hours. Sensitivity declines with time. If CT is negative and suspicion of SAH remains on clinical grounds, then lumbar puncture is indicated as long as there is no coagulation abnormality and no suspicion of dangerously increased intracranial pressure. Erythrocytes lyse and disappear from the CSF in 3 to 7 days following SAH. Xanthochromia (yellow pigmentation from heme breakdown products) persists in the CSF for 2 weeks following SAH in virtually all cases and in up to 70% for as long as 3 weeks. The most sensitive way to detect xanthochromia is by spectrophotometric analysis; visual inspection alone is less sensitive.

53. A: Lipohyalinosis is a specific condition of small vessels that leads to lacunar stroke by predisposing to microatheroma and thrombosis. Whether cardioembolism is ever a cause of lacunar infarct is in dispute; it is certainly not the underlying pathologic process in most cases. Lacunae are generally not hemorrhagic, and vascular malformations do not cause lacunar infarcts.

54. D: Hypertension is the greatest risk factor for lacunar infarct; cigarette smoking, advanced age, hyperlipidemia, and diabetes are lesser risk factors Lacunar infarcts are tiny areas of ischemic necrosis caused by occlusion of small penetrating arteries. Although lacunar infarcts are small, their symptoms may be major because of their strategic location in "eloquent" areas of the brain and brainstem. Lacunar strokes account for approximately 25% of ischemic strokes and fall into 5 classic syndromes first chronicled by C. Miller Fisher. These include pure motor hemiparesis, ataxic hemiparesis, dysarthria/clumsy hand syndrome, pure sensory stroke, and mixed sensorimotor stroke.

55. C: Stress and dietary triggers are relevant for some but not all migraineurs. No patient with daily headache of any etiology will respond to pharmacologic prophylaxis in the presence of on-going daily analgesic therapy because of analgesic rebound syndrome. Most patients are reluctant to discontinue analgesics, and it is important to explain the analgesic rebound syndrome carefully and supportively. Analgesics should be changed to a time-contingent schedule and gradually tapered rather than abruptly discontinued. Physical medicine is the mainstay of therapy for patients with myofascial pain syndromes, including headache, but not for migraine.

56. A: There are many pain-sensitive structures in the head and neck, giving rise to multiple anatomic causes for headache, but the brain parenchyma itself is not a pain-sensitive tissue.

57. C: The triptans, which are selective (5-HT) serotonin receptor antagonists, are available in oral, sublingual, nasal, and subcutaneously injectable forms and constitute the most effective form of acute therapy for most moderately severe or severe migraines as long as there is no medical contraindication, such as hypertension or coronary artery disease. Ergot alkaloids, such as ergotamine tartrate and dihydroergotamine, are less selective and often cause more side effects than the triptans. Tricyclic antidepressants, beta-blockers, and anticonvulsant medications can all be used effectively to reduce the frequency of migraine attacks but are not useful for interrupting an established attack.

58. B: Many patients with cluster headaches that break through prophylactic treatment can manage breakthrough headaches at home by starting oxygen inhalation promptly at the onset of headache. This is a practical approach for patients whose headaches generally occur at night and awaken them from sleep when they are at home and close to their oxygen supply. Since cluster headaches escalate rapidly to peak intensity, early intervention is important and parenteral routes of medication administration are often preferable. Triptans can be taken intranasally or subcutaneously; dihydroergotamine (DHE) can be taken intranasally, subcutaneously or intramuscularly; and lidocaine can be taken intranasally.

59. C: A patient presenting with dull headache with superimposed icepick sensations and jaw claudication accompanied by elevated ESR has classic symptoms of giant cell arteritis. While false-negative biopsies do occur, nonetheless, temporal artery biopsy is essential. The most severe consequence of untreated giant cell arteritis is blindness due to ischemic optic neuropathy, and this is preventable with corticosteroid therapy. Since effective treatment requires high doses given over at least 4-6 weeks, treatment should not be undertaken without as much diagnostic evidence as possible. Although there is some evidence that loss of vision is unlikely in the absence of a positive temporal artery biopsy, many physicians will treat in the absence of a positive biopsy if the other clinical evidence is overwhelming, because the risk of withholding treatment is irreversible loss of vision. Once vision is lost, corticosteroid treatment will not restore it. Central retinal artery occlusion can also cause loss of vision in patients with giant cell arteritis.

60: D: Cigarette smoking is a perpetuating factor for some patients with common migraine, migraine with aura, and tension-type headache, but for nearly all patients with cluster headache, cigarette smoking, if present, is an insurmountable obstacle to effective harmacologic prophylaxis.

61. D: The use of prophylactic antibiotics for patients with CSF leak due to basal skull fracture is a matter of controversy and is subject to clinical judgment. On the one hand, the risk of meningitis is substantial, and meningitis is a serious infection; on the other hand, most patients, even untreated, do not develop meningitis, and prophylactic antibiotics may increase the risk of even more serious infection with resistant organisms. Most CSF leaks resolve spontaneously within 7 to 10 days. The bones at the base of the skull are delicate, and the meninges are closely applied to the inner surface of the skull, so CSF leak is not an uncommon complication of basal skull fracture.

62. A: This child is presenting in classic manner with an evolving epidural hematoma. Most epidural hematomas occur in children and young adults, in whom the attachment of the dura to the undersurface of the skull is less secure than in older adults. Most epidural hematomas are of arterial origin, usually the middle meningeal artery or one of its branches. Blood in the epidural space is more likely to cause clinically significant mass effect on the brain than an equivalent volume of blood in the subdural space, and patients can deteriorate rapidly and even progress to transtentorial herniation without prompt intervention. The most efficient way to make the diagnosis is by non-contrast CT scan of the brain, which will clearly show a biconvex hyperintense hematoma. Surgical evacuation is indicated if the clinical picture is deteriorating and/or if the hematoma is 1 cm or more in greatest diameter.

63. B: Epidural hematomas are usually (85%) arterial in origin, but subdural hematomas usually result from tearing of bridging veins. Contusion is a less common cause of subdural hematoma. It is always prudent to look for an underlying coagulopathy in the presence of a subdural hematoma, but in most cases, none will be found.
Matrix classification: 1

64. D: Comment: Definitive diagnosis of DAI requires microscopic examination of brain tissue. The shearing injury caused by acceleration/deceleration forces generally causes microscopic changes that are not evident at all on CT. MRI is usually also normal, although there may be tiny focal abnormalities. In practice, diagnosis of DAI is a clinical diagnosis.

65. B: The brain has very limited reserves and cannot tolerate hypoxia for more than a few minutes. Even PaO2 under 90% predicts a poor neurologic outcome. The goal of ventilator management is to provide adequate oxygen to the brain en route to the hospital. Management of PaCO2 is also important, but the goal is simply to keep the PaCO2 in the physiologic range. Since the effect of hypocapnia is short-lived at best, there is no advantage to lowering the PaCO preemptively. Ventilator-induced hypocapnia should be reserved for short-term use when intracranial pressure is believed to be dangerously increased and herniation is likely without intervention. Even then, hypocapnia is not a definitive solution, and surgical intervention should be at hand. Oxygen toxicity is a longer-term consideration. The immediate need in this setting is to maintain adequate oxygen delivery to the brain, even if it is necessary to use 100% O2.

66. A: This patient is presenting signs of autonomic dysfunction syndrome (ADS,) sometimes known as autonomic storm. Sometimes this autonomic dysfunction is episodic, occurring transiently in response to stimuli such as airway suctioning. Additional signs may include diaphoresis, cardiac arrhythmias, pupillary dilatation, decorticate posturing, or decerebrate posturing. This syndrome results from damage to the hypothalamus and/or brainstem structures that regulate autonomic function, and/or to the areas of cortex that influence neural activity in the hypothalamus and/or brainstem. In addition to managing the autonomic function of each organ system involved, it is possible to treat the syndrome as a whole with a variety of pharmacologic approaches, the most common of which is careful titration of intravenous morphine sulfate. Other approaches include beta-blockers, clonidine, dantrolene, and bromocriptine. Prompt recognition and intervention to treat ADS are important to prevent secondary brain injury (usually resulting from fever) as well as other end-organ damage, such as pulmonary edema or myocardial injury.

67. B: The incidence of lateral transtentorial herniation due to cerebral edema peaks at 72 hours following injury. The most obviou sign is a dilated, nonreactive pupil, but a sluggishly reacting oval pupil often precedes this more dramatic papillary change. In either case, the change reflects compression of the ipsilateral oculomotor nerve by the herniating cerebral hemisphere.

68. C: Infection is the greatest risk of an intraventricular catheter, so the drain should be opened only at intervals and for no more than 5 minutes at a time. Cerebrospinal fluid should be drained extremely slowly to avoid sudden shifts in intracranial pressure.

69. D: If there is even suspicion of a basal skull fracture, the patient should not be suctioned through the nose. When the fragile bones at the base of the skull sustain fractures, there is often tearing of the closely applied dura. The catheter could penetrate a tear in the dura and introduce infection into the central nervous system. When a basal fracture involves the middle fossa, there is also danger of introducing infection via the ear. A good precaution is to place sterile cotton over the nares or external auditory canal, depending on the site of the fracture, and to change the cotton frequently.

70. B: Until spine imaging has been completed and injury that could compromise the spinal cord excluded, the patient must remain on the backboard. The physician makes the determination of when the patient can safely be removed from the board. As time passes, the risk of decubitus ulcers increases. The nurse should note the passage of time and inform the other members of the team as time passes and the risk of soft tissue damage increases.

71. B: With spinal cord injury at any level, bladder reflexes are likely to be lost, and the patient should be assumed to have an atonic bladder on admission. After 24-48 hours, it is time to remove the indwelling catheter and begin a program of intermittent catheterization. Intermittent catheterization performed with aseptic technique carries less risk of infection than an indwelling catheter. Antibiotics are not necessary unless a urinary tract infection actually ensues.

72. D: Comment: Following spinal cord injury, peristalsis stops and paralytic ileus ensues. The abdomen will become distended, even to the point of compromising breathing, if there is no avenue of decompression. Depending on when peristalsis returns, and depending on other factors such as the patient's level of consciousness, it may be necessary to provide total parenteral nutrition, but this is not an immediate consideration in the emergency department.

73. C: This patient is experiencing autonomic dysreflexia (AD). This is a condition of massive sympathetic outflow from the cord below the level of the lesion. This may occur spontaneously but more often it results from noxious peripheral stimulation, and the most common underlying condition is distention of the bladder. If the patient has graduated to a program of intermittent catheterization, the bladder should be catheterized immediately as soon as evidence of AD is detected. Other peripheral stimuli capable of inciting AD include bladder infection, kidney stones, bowel impaction, and cutaneous injuries of any kind, such as decubitus ulcers or even ingrown toenails. The bladder is the first place to check. Once the inciting stimulus is removed, antihypertensive drugs may still be needed. The hypertension associated with AD can be extreme and can lead to hemorrhagic stroke, subarachnoid hemorrhage, or damage to other end-0rgans, including the retina and the myocardium. AD is therefore to be treated as a medical emergency.

74. A: The radial nerve is most vulnerable to trauma as it wraps around the humerus, so a fractured humerus is the most common cause of radial nerve injury. Radial fractures are less likely to damage the radial nerve but may do so in some cases. Shoulder dislocation can injure the median nerve.

75. D: This patient has bilateral carpal tunnel syndrome caused by compression of the median nerves in the very narrow carpal tunnel, which is bound superiorly by the transverse carpal ligaments and inferolaterally by the carpal bones. These structures are relatively inflexible, so if

edema accumulates in the carpal tunnel, it will compress the median nerve within it. This occurs commonly during pregnancy and almost always resolves spontaneously in the weeks following delivery. Conservative measures are sufficient unless the patient develops prominent motor symptoms or disabling pain. While she will benefit from elevating her hands slightly whenever she can, including during sleep, the peripheral nerve injury associated with draping the upper arm over a chair or misusing crutches is radial palsy, and this patient has signs of carpal tunnel syndrome, not radial palsy.

76. A: The male to female ratio in patients with chronic subdural hematoma is 2:1. The average age of patients with chronic SDH is 69. Alcoholism predisposes an individual to SDH not only by increasing the risk of trauma, but also via cerebral atrophy, which leaves the subdural space slightly expanded, stretching the bridging veins. While trauma is a risk factor for SDH, the trauma is often surprisingly mild, and up to 25% of SDH patients have no known antecedent history of trauma. Coagulopathy is also a risk factor for chronic SDH. SDH may mimic other neurologic syndromes that are prevalent in elderly populations, including dementia and Parkinson's disease.

77. B: This patient has peroneal nerve palsy. The peroneal nerve receives input from roots L4, L5, S1, and S2 via the sciatic nerve. It is vulnerable to pressure injury as it passes behind the head of the fibula. Nursing care of the immobilized patient includes protection of this vulnerable site. Recovery from peroneal palsy due to pressure injury takes several months, during which the patient will need splints or other protective measures to prevent further injury associated with foot drop. Most patients will experience moderately severe to severe neuropathic pain, which responds partially to a range of medications, including anticonvulsants, tricyclic antidepressants, and opioid analgesics.

78. D: Cerebrospinal fluid (CSF) accumulates in the subdural space when a tear in the underlying meninges allows CSF to escape, forming a hygroma. The symptoms resemble those of subdural hematoma, including the pace of presentation, and headache is prominent. The lesion remains unilateral and may become encapsulated.

79. B: The primary goal of a bowel management regimen is to allow the patient to have a soft, formed stool every 1 to 3 days. While laxative overuse is to be avoided, it is reasonable to use mild laxatives when necessary. Stool softeners, bulk-forming agents, and suppositories can also be helpful. The patient should follow a diet with ample roughage. While regularity in the stimuli that affect bowel function – such as meals, medications, suppositories, and visits to the bathroom – should follow a regular schedule as much as possible, it really doesn't matter when the patient eventually defecates. In the early stages of spinal cord injury, Valsalva is to be avoided because of the risk of autonomic dysreflexia. By the time the acute phase has passed, it will be clear if the patient can or cannot tolerate gentle Valsalva; if he can, then this method of assisting a bowel movement should be encouraged.

80. D: Rapid normalization of the serum sodium is not necessary as the neurologic sequelae of the electrolyte imbalance will begin to improve even before full correction is achieved. Rapid normalization also carries the risk of central pontine myelinolysis, which is an irreversible central nervous system injury with devastating consequences. Hypertonic saline and furosemide can be used cautiously to begin to reverse the hyponatremia, after which further normalization should be

accomplished through fluid restriction. Demeclocycline is of benefit in the chronic, but not acute, management of hyponatremia due to syndrome of inappropriate antidiuretic hormone (SIADH) but not in the management of psychogenic polydipsia, which is the likely cause of water intoxication in this patient whose diagnosis of schizophrenia is known to the emergency department.

In addition to central pontine myelinolysis, other potential complications of hypertonic saline include intravascular hemolysis, pulmonary edema, and hypokalemia.

81. B: In the setting of neurologic care units, it is still important to remain alert for non-neurologic problems, particularly in the face of trauma. Pain on straight leg raising is suggestive of herniated nucleus pulposus, but pain on passive flexion of the hip suggests a hip fracture.

82. D: Spinal cord edema frequently develops during the acute phase following spinal cord injury. The spinal cord does not tolerate edema well, and a patient who has been breathing well could rapidly develop respiratory compromise if edema begins to affect higher segments of the cord that innervate the intercostal muscles and diaphragm. It is also important to monitor the patient for evidence of peripheral skeletal injuries or internal visceral injuries that may be masked by sensory deficits caused by the spinal cord injury.

83. D: Comment: The most common cause of low back pain in middle-aged persons is lumbar strain. In the absence of symptoms or signs of nerve root compromise, it is not necessary to investigate the possibility of disc herniation. Spinal stenosis is mostly a condition of adults over age 50. Spondylolysis is a defect in the pars articularis, most commonly in the lower lumbar vertebrae. It is usually caused by stress injury in young people who over train in various sports or engage in contact sports, especially football.

84. A: Comment: In the absence of motor impairment, most patients with carpal tunnel do not require surgery. Treatment consists of managing any underlying medical condition such as diabetes, thyroid disease, or arthritis and use of wrist splints, and physical therapy. Nonsteroidal anti-inflammatory medications, diuretics, and corticosteroids may be used if there is no contraindication, and steroid injection into the wrist is an option.

85. B: Erb's palsy is an injury of the upper brachial plexus during childbirth. The affected infant has weakness of the affected arm and tends to hold the forearm pronated with the wrist flexed. The injury is caused by stretching the brachial plexus during delivery. Shoulder dystocia makes such stretching more likely, as does precipitous delivery. Larger babies are more at risk; hence gestational diabetes is a risk factor. Premature delivery is not a risk factor.

86. A: Most babies with Erb's palsy have stretch injury without nerve avulsion and recover well within 3 to 6 months. During this time, it is important to keep the joints mobilized with passive range of motion exercises and to protect the baby from injury. These measures are equally important for those babies who do not recover and go on to surgical intervention. If the Erb's palsy is attributable to a maternal condition that is likely to be present during a subsequent pregnancy, such as a narrow pelvis, then the mother should be made aware of the risk in subsequent pregnancies so that she can consider her approach to childbirth, but this is not the most important

or most immediate concern during the first few days of the life of the new infant under consideration. Erb's palsy, like any birth injury, often raises questions of liability, but this is also not the immediate nursing concern when the parents are about to take a baby with Erb's palsy home from the hospital.

87. D: Facial fractures are often associated with anosmia as the olfactory fibers are easily injured as they traverse the cribriform plate. Anosmia puts patients at risk for poisoning by ingesting spoiled food. Other cranial nerve injuries are associated with basal skull fractures, but these are less frequent, and those that would affect the muscles of mastication or swallowing would have become evident prior to discharge.

88. A: An unconscious patient without a diagnosis may have had head trauma as the cause of loss of consciousness or may have sustained head trauma as a result of losing consciousness for some other reason. In either case, it is important to be alert to signs of possible basal skull fracture. Basal fracture in the middle fossa manifests as hemotympanum or otorrhea. Otoscopic examination alone will not yield information about vestibular dysfunction, although vestibular dysfunction can result from basal fractures. Battle's sign (ecchymosis over the temporal bone) does not develop for 12 to 24 hours following fracture.

89. D: Barbiturates protect the brain by lowering cerebral metabolic demand, inhibiting lipid damage, and allowing reducing cerebral blood flow, especially to areas of lower metabolism. Hyperventilation is a short-term intervention that temporarily reduces cerebral blood flow by lowering $PaCO2$, which triggers vasoconstriction. Hyperventilation is not without risks and should not be undertaken unless a more definitive approach, such as ventriculostomy, is imminent. Hypertonic saline temporarily reduces intracranial pressure by reducing brain water content. Hypertonic saline carries risks, including central pontine myelinolysis, intravascular hemorrhage, and hypokalemia. Glucocorticoids are widely used to treat edema and inflammation in various parts of the body, but studies show that they are actually not effective in treating cerebral edema. Because they are not effective and because they carry multiple risks, including infection, hyperglycemia, osteoporosis, and cataracts, glucocorticoids are contraindicated for the treatment of increased intracranial pressure.

90. A: Excessively rapid infusion of phenytoin can induce hypotension and cardiac arrhythmia. There is less risk of hypotension with fosphenytoin, which is preferred for patients who are not hemodynamically stable. Rate of infusion does not influence allergic reaction, but every precaution should be taken not to administer a drug to which a patient is allergic. Phenytoin can cause endovascular irritation because of the alkalinity of the solution; the best precaution to avoid vein irritation is to flush with normal saline after the infusion is finished. Soft tissue damage is not a risk; phenytoin can be given intramuscularly.

91. A: Glucose-containing IV fluids can contribute to neurotoxic acidosis. The risk of cerebral edema is associated with hypotonic IV fluids. Hypokalemia is avoided simply by monitoring electrolytes and providing sufficient potassium in the IV fluid.

92. D: As children grow, the volume of distribution of anticonvulsant drugs will increase. This factor alone will require dose adjustment throughout childhood and adolescence. While noncompliance can be an issue, it is important not to attribute low serum drug levels to noncompliance when normal growth accounts for the change. Serum concentrations of anticonvulsant medications will also be affected by many, if not most, other medications taken concurrently and by hormonal changes.

93. C: Dextrose can cause phenytoin to precipitate out of solution.

94. C: The cachexia suggests that this patient has chronically poor nutrition, possibly related to alcoholism. He is probably thiamine deficient which places him at risk for Wernicke-Korsakoff' syndrome; although recovery from this condition is possible, prevention is the best approach. There is no harm in giving thiamine, so it should be given on the basis of this suspicion alone. It is best to give the thiamine before the patient receives any intravenous fluids containing dextrose, as glucose can precipitate encephalopathy in a thiamine-deficient patient.

Wernicke's encephalopathy is not the same as Wernicke's aphasia. Wernicke's encephalopathy presents with globally depressed cognition, abnormalities of eye movements, and gait ataxia. Untreated, Wernicke's encephalopathy may progress to Korsakoff's psychosis, which consists of retrograde and anterograde amnesia with confabulation. While Wernicke-Korsakoff syndrome is classically associated with alcoholism, it can be caused by any condition that chronically interferes with nutrition, such as AIDS or hyperemesis.

The recommended thiamine dosage in the emergency room is 250 mg intramuscularly. As the patient recovers, he should receive 100 mg orally every day. Physicians often overlook thiamine replacement, and some are reluctant to give intramuscular thiamine in the emergency room because of concern about anaphylactic reactions. In fact, the incidence of anaphylactic reaction to thiamine is less than that of anaphylactic reaction to penicillin.

95. B: This child has typical absence seizures, a primary generalized seizure type in which spells are often so subtle as to escape notice altogether even when parents and teachers are quite observant. The principal manifestation is often underperformance in school, which is often incorrectly attributed to inattentiveness. Seizures can be very frequent – hundreds of times per day – causing the child to miss a great deal of what transpires in the classroom. The characteristic EEG signature consists of regular, generalized 3-Hz spike-wave complexes that come and go abruptly.

In atypical absence, the spells last longer, have less abrupt onset and offset, and include more obvious motor elements. The signature EEG abnormality is an irregular 2.5-Hz or less spike-wave pattern.

Absence seizures are usually quite easily controlled with medication – valproic acid, ethosuximide, or lamotrigine – and cognitive function improves dramatically. Most children with absence outgrow their spells by early adulthood. Those who do not outgrow them often go on to experience additional seizure types later in life.

96. A: Cognitive impairment affects at least 60% of persons with multiple sclerosis. The type and degree of cognitive impairment varies considerably from individual to individual. The picture is rarely that of a true dementia in which cognitive function is globally affected. Rather, a particular skill is compromised, such as short-term memory or multi-tasking. Early treatment with disease-modifying agents can forestall cognitive impairment, and this is among the most persuasive arguments for early treatment.

97. D: Comment: Surgery does not cure most primary malignant brain tumors. There is evidence, however, that survival is improved in proportion to the amount of malignant tissue that is removed. Unlike malignancies of other organ systems, primary malignant tumors of the brain rarely metastasize outside the central nervous system. There are many ways to control increased intracranial pressure, and the choice of approach is determined by the numerous variables of the particular clinical situation.

98. A: The primary advantage for gamma-knife treatment is its specificity. It can target malignant tissue with great precision, thus, sparing surrounding normal tissues. However, this advantage also constitutes a potential disadvantage when malignant infiltration escapes imaging as the radiation beam will not be directed to the undetected infiltrating margins of the tumor. For this reason, gamma-knife is most effective when deployed to treat circumscribed lesions of 4 cm or less in greatest diameter. No treatment approach to malignant brain tumors is curative.

99. D: f an oligodendroglioma is marked by allelic loss of heterozygosity in the 1p and 19q chromosome arms, then it will have a nearly 100% likelihood of responding to either chemotherapy alone or chemotherapy in combination with radiation therapy. Without this marker, response rate ranges from 15% to 30%. Response does not mean cure, however.

Chemotherapy with temozolomide combined with radiation therapy has also become standard of care for patients with glioblastoma multiforme.

100. B: The incidence of medulloblastoma, like that of pilocytic astrocytoma and germ cell tumors, decreases with age. The incidence of most other brain tumors, both benign and malignant, increases with age.

101. B: If a tumor that is histologically benign is located in such a way as to be surgically inaccessible or in a location where surgery is contraindicated because it would cause unacceptable neurologic deficits, then it is benign only in the histological sense, but can still be incurable. Since most brain tumors are not cured by radiation or chemotherapy in the absence of surgical debulking, most inoperable brain tumors are fatal.

102. D: Neurons and glial cells both derive from the neural tube, which in turn derives from the ectodermal (outer) layer of the embryo. The glial cells include astrocytes, ligodendrocytes, and ependymal cells, all of which are capable of malignant transformation, giving rise to astrocytomas, oligodendrogliomas, and ependymomas. Each of these tumor types is further classified according to histologic characteristics.

The anterior pituitary is derived from the surface ectoderm, while the posterior pituitary is derived from the neuroectoderm. Pituitary adenomas are tumors of the anterior pituitary gland.

103. B: Acoustic neuroma is a benign neoplasm of cranial nerve VIII; metastasis is not a concern. Smaller tumors can be removed completely, but when hearing has been lost, it is rarely restored. It is, however, a realistic goal of surgery to prevent permanent palsy of cranial nerve VII, which is in close proximity to cranial nerve VIII in the cerebellopontine angle. When an acoustic neuroma is too large to be removed surgically, or if the patient is not a suitable surgical candidate for independent medical reasons, then radiation therapy can reduce the size of the tumor and slow its subsequent growth.

A more accurate name for this tumor is vestibular Schwannoma, because it actually involves the vestibular portion of cranial nerve VIII, and the cell of origin is the Schwann cell, which is responsible for forming the nerve's myelin sheath.

104. A: Hemangioblastoma is a benign vascular neoplasm that occurs almost exclusively in the central nervous system, most frequently in the posterior fossa, where it constitutes 8-10% of all neoplasms. The presenting symptoms of hemangioblastoma are usually referable to cerebellar dysfunction and may include gait and appendicular ataxia. The neoplasm may also present with headache and other symptoms related to obstruction of the ventricular system and associated increased intracranial pressure.

105. C: This patient has a cerebellar hemangioma. The polycythemia is present as a paraneoplastic phenomenon, which is frequently associated with this tumor type. The associated adrenal tumor identifies this patient as having von Hippel-Lindau disease. About 25% of patients with hemangioblastoma have this autosomal dominant syndrome, which may include retinal angiomatosis, and tumors of the adrenal glands and kidneys in addition to the central nervous system hemangioma. Family members should be offered genetic screening.

106. D: Methotrexate can cause toxicity to virtually every organ system, particularly the liver and lungs. Salicylates and NSAIDs displace methotrexate from serum albumin,ncreasing the free drug concentration, while simultaneously inhibiting renal tubular excretion of the drug.

107. A: In the absence of immunosuppression, primary central nervous system lymphoma (PCNSL) is not a common malignancy, accounting for fewer than 2% of central nervous system neoplasms. PCNSL occurs in 6-20% of HIV-infected persons, however. Among HIV-infected patients with PCNSL, intravenous drug use constitutes a significant risk factor. In addition to HIV, other conditions associated with immunosuppression increase the risk of PCNSL. These include immunosuppression following organ transplant and prolonged use of glucocorticoids to treat autoimmune disorders.

108. D: Neurofibromatosis is inherited in an autosomal dominant fashion. The precise location of the abnormal genes for neurofibromatosis type 1 (NF1) and neurofibromatosis type 2 (NF2) has been identified. A substantial percentage of patients with neurofibromatosis have the disorder on

the basis of a spontaneous mutation; although these patients come from families without neurofibromatosis, they can pass it on to their children with 50% risk for each mating.

109. A: Comment: Von-Hippel Lindau disease is an autosomal recessive disorder characterized by multiple benign hemangiomas of the central nervous system. Other types of tumors, including hypernephroma, angioma, and pheochromocytoma, can affect the kidney and adrenal glands in patients with von-Hippel Lindau disease. Management is generally surgical, based on location and mass effect of the tumors. Targeted radiation can also be used.

110. B: At least 90% of meningiomas are benign tumors. Some are found near the site of head trauma, but a causal relationship is not fully established. There is also some suggestion of a viral etiology in some cases, but no clear causal relationship is established for this factor either. Radiation exposure, however, is a clear risk factor for meningioma. Meningiomas in radiation-exposed individuals tend to be more aggressive than meningiomas that arise in the absence of radiation exposure. Asbestos exposure is a risk factor for mesothelioma, but not for meningioma.

111. B: The scenario described constitutes pituitary apoplexy in which the benign tumor either hemorrhages into itself or outgrows its blood supply, causing infarction and adjacent edema. Pituitary apoplexy is a surgical emergency. Because the patient will likely have endocrine dysfunction, endocrine support, especially with glucocorticoids, will be necessary.

112. A: Many patients with pituitary adenomas are unable to produce adequate levels of thyroid hormone and/or glucocorticoids to meet the challenge of surgical trauma. Subjecting these patients to surgery without giving them the necessary hormonal support exposes them to increased risk, even fatality.

113. C: Bilateral hemianopia results from pressure on the optic chiasm, classically from a pituitary adenoma growing upward out of the sella turcica.

114. B: Medical treatment for a cholesteatoma is almost never effective. A cholesteatoma is a collection of squamous cells trapped within the temporal bone. The condition is either congenital or acquired. Although the cells are benign, as they grow, they cause bony erosion and can cause mass effect on the brain at the base of the skull, as well as causing conductive hearing loss. Cholesteatomas can form abscesses and can lead to meningitis. While histologically benign, cholesteatomas can be fatal. When they become infected, antibiotics almost never fully eradicate the infection, because cholesteatomas have no blood supply of their own. Antibiotics may reach the periphery of the lesion, but infection in its interior is not eradicated by antibiotics. Surgical treatment is mandatory for every cholesteatoma unless there is an overwhelming medical contraindication to surgery that cannot be eliminated or overcome.

115. D: Radiosurgery is a noninvasive technique that uses CT and/or MRI images in the operating room to direct radiation therapy directly to the metastases, sparing the brain as a whole. Survival with this technique is superior to survival with whole brain radiation and surgery. Chemotherapy is generally impractical for brain tumors, although novel delivery systems may enhance the effectiveness of chemotherapy in some cases.

116. A: Intramedullary spinal tumors are rare compared with brain tumors. Most are benign and can be resected completely for a cure. Surgery should be the first-line therapy in most cases, unless there is an unreversed coagulopathy or severe infection, or some other absolute medical contraindication to surgery. Most intramedullary spinal cord tumors arise from non-neural cells. Although most of these tumors are histologically benign, their mass effect can produce overwhelming often irreversible neurologic deficits. Surgery should be the first-line therapy and should be offered without delay.

117. D: Chemotherapy is still considered experimental for the treatment of primary spinal cord tumors. Most spinal cord tumors are slow growing and can be cured with surgical excision. Radiation therapy is a second line of treatment, and chemotherapy is investigational.

118. B: It is correct that the metabolism of the halogenated volatile anesthetics is inhibited by NO, and it is correct that the halogenated volatile anesthetics can provoke cardiac arrhythmias by blocking membrane ion channels, but these are considerations that apply to the use of these agents in any situation. The consideration that is specifically and uniquely important in spinal surgery is that these agents can interfere with somatosensory evoked potential monitoring, which has become a standard part of operating room protocol for surgeries involving the spinal cord.

119. A: Patients with significant neurologic deficit have a poor prognosis for neurologic recovery following surgery, even if the tumor is entirely resected. This is the main argument for early surgical intervention, even if the tumor is thought to be histologically benign. Presence of a syrinx is actually a positive prognostic sign, probably because syrinx formation is usually associated with noninfiltrating neoplasms. Surgical outcome does not vary with sex. Tumors involving the cervical and upper thoracic cord have, in general, a worse neurologic prognosis than tumors of the lumbar cord.

120. C: The blood circulation is the most common route of metastasis into the central nervous system. Malignancies that have excellent access to the circulation, such as lung cancers, are particularly likely to metastasize to the brain. Meningeal carcinomatosis (metastatic cells in the cerebrospinal fluid) is characteristic of acute lymphocytic leukemia and non-Hodgkin's lymphoma, but overall, the hematogenous route is the most common mode of entry of metastases into the central nervous system.

121. B: The neuronal inflammation associated with Bell's palsy has been attributed to viral infection, and Herpes simplex viral particles have been isolated from neurons of patients with Bell's palsy. On this basis, it has been suggested that antiviral medication should confer some additional benefit when added to steroid therapy, which does improve outcomes in Bell's palsy compared with placebo. Recent guidelines published by the American Academy of Neurology state that acyclovir combined with steroid medication is "possibly effective" in treating Bell's palsy. Nonetheless, a meta-analysis of six trials comprising 1145 patients showed no advantage of antiviral medication plus steroids over steroids alone in terms of motor outcome. These results were consistent regardless of the degree of paralysis at the height of the symptoms and across all antivirals used (acyclovir, famciclovir, valacyclovir.)

122. D: Chiari malformation (classified into types I, II, III and IV) is characterized by malformation of the bones at the base of the skull with varying degrees of downward displacement of the cerebellar tonsils into the foramen magnum, causing pressure on brainstem structures. Some types of Chiari malformation are accompanied by syringomyelia. Headache is the classic presenting symptom. Other symptoms are referable to pressure on brainstem and cervical cord structures. The differential diagnosis prominently includes multiple sclerosis, as well as structural lesions of the cervical cord. Symptoms referable to cortical irritation, such as seizures, are not part of the clinical picture.

123. D: Comment: Cerebral palsy has been classically attributed to hypoxia sustained during delivery, but studies find an association between childbirth complications and cerebral palsy in no more than 10% of cases. Just as the clinical picture is highly variable, so too are the potential causes, which include prematurity, occult viral or bacterial infection during pregnancy, Rh incompatibility, uncontrolled maternal diabetes, maternal nutritional deficiencies, X-ray exposure, maternal anemia, and jaundice. Many of the brain injuries that cause cerebral palsy occur during intrauterine development, well in advance of delivery. Thus, not only is meticulous obstetric care essential to prevent cerebral palsy; so too is comprehensive prenatal care.

124. A: Most children and adults with cerebral palsy will need some medication at some point to treat their spasticity, but no pharmacologic regimen will provide optimal results in the absence of physical therapy to prevent contractures and promote flexibility. The family, and eventually the patient himself or herself, can take primary responsibility for maintenance physical therapy. If oral medication is poorly tolerated – side effects commonly include somnolence and nausea – then other routes of medication delivery can be considered, such as intrathecal baclofen or injections of botulinum toxin.

125. C: Spina bifida is a developmental disorder involving incomplete closure of the neural tube. It is, therefore, determined early in the course of prenatal life, well before birth. In addition to pre-pregnancy maternal obesity, maternal diabetes, and maternal folic acid deficiency, other risk factors include maternal hyperthermia in early pregnancy, and certain medications, particularly valproic acid. The risk of spinal bifida increases in families with spina bifida, and the incidence is higher among persons of northern European and Hispanic descent than among those of Asian and African descent, and higher among females than among males.

126. A: Spina bifida is a defect of neural tube closure. If the defect is minor, involving only a portion of a vertebral body, it is called spinal bifida occulta and is generally asymptomatic, coming to attention only incidentally when X-rays are obtained for an independent reason. More frequently, the spinal cord and its covering membranes are exposed through the defect, and this condition is myelomeningocele. Many children with spina bifida and myelomeningocele also have hydrocephalus and some develop syringomyelia.
Matrix classification: 6

127. B: Alpha-fetoprotein of the yolk sac and later of the fetal liver is related to the protein albumin. Elevated maternal levels are a marker for neural tube defects, including spina bifida. Abnormally low levels are associated with Down's syndrome. In adults, alpha-fetoprotein is produced in trace

amounts. Elevated adult levels are associated with various malignancies, including hepatocellular carcinoma, ovarian carcinoma, testicular carcinoma, and malignant teratoma.

128. D: Occasionally, a tiny asymptomatic syrinx may be found on MRI performed for an independent reason; in these cases, the syrinx is often of no clinical significance and can reasonably be monitored without intervention unless symptoms develop or the syrinx is observed to enlarge over time. Symptomatic syringomyelia, however, is nearly always slowly progressive. Surgery halts progression in many cases but usually fails to reverse established neurologic disability, so early intervention is preferable. The symptoms of syringomyelia overlap with those of multiple sclerosis, which usually has an early course characterized by exacerbations and remissions. MRI easily distinguishes between these two conditions.

129. C: Most patients with symptomatic syringomyelia experience spasticity, weakness, and pain. The spasticity may mask the true degree of weakness present, and overtreating the spasticity may unmask weakness to such an extent that the patient loses important motor function. Some patients with syringomyelia rely on their spasticity to be able to stand with support to carry on important functions such as dressing, preparing food, or folding clothes. Treatment of spasticity in these patients needs to be balanced so as not to inadvertently increase weakness.

On the other hand, spasticity often increases pain, and treating spasticity may contribute to improved pain control. Balancing the management of spasticity, weakness, and pain, therefore, requires excellent communication and clinical finesse. Sensory function other than pain is not affected by treatment for spasticity.

130. A: The frontotemporal dementias are characterized by aphasia out of proportion to other cognitive difficulties. Personality changes may be prominent as well, leading to incorrect psychiatric diagnoses. Impaired recent memory out of proportion to remote memory is a characteristic of Alzheimer's disease.

131. A: Huperzine A acts as a cholinesterase inhibitor. It should not be taken concurrently with prescription cholinesterase inhibitors (donepezil, rivastigmine, and galantamine) because of the increased risk of toxic side effects. Memantine is not a cholinesterase inhibitor – it is a glutamatergic NMDA receptor antagonist and a dopamine D2 receptor agonist – and can be taken concurrently with huperzine A. Ginkgo biloba is contraindicated in the presence of anticoagulants. It is always important to take a complete drug history, including nonprescription preparations, in order to be aware of possible drug interactions.

132. B: Cholinesterase inhibitors (donepezil, rivastigmine, galantamine) increase levels of acetylcholine in subcortical regions. In a very small subset of patients with Alzheimer's disease, these medications may dramatically, although not permanently, reverse some cognitive deficits. For the most part, however, the most that can be expected is for about half of Alzheimer's disease patients treated to respond by having symptom progression delayed for 6 to 12 months.

133. B: The best strategy to insure that a patient in the middle stages of Alzheimer's disease executes complex instructions correctly is to provide both verbal and nonverbal cues

simultaneously, such as handing the patient his toothbrush and then placing a cup for rinsing his mouth next to him, while saying, "First brush your teeth, and then rinse." Written lists are not likely to be helpful after the early stage of the disease, as the patient may forget to even look at the list and will eventually experience deterioration in his ability to read. Reading should be encouraged early in the course of the disease, as long as it has a positive effect, but it should not be relied upon as a memory device, especially as the disease progresses. One should speak clearly but softly. Object cues (objects placed in the environment as a visual reminder to take a necessary action) are helpful in the early stages of the disease, but they fail to prompt the desired response as the disease progresses.

134. D: As Alzheimer's disease progresses, patients have increasing difficulty responding to open-ended questions, but nearly everyone still appreciates the feeling of being able to make choices whenever possible. Offering the person a choice between two reasonable alternatives removes the overwhelming aspect of an open-ended question that requires more memory, imagination, and vocabulary than he may be able to bring to bear while still preserving as much autonomy as possible.

135. D: Comment: It is best not to comment on the reality of the experience unless the patient himself questions it. Antipsychotic medications should be avoided unless behavioral interventions fail and the hallucinations or delusions are very distressing to the patient or give rise to very disruptive behaviors. Antipsychotic medications carry greater risks of side effects, including stroke, metabolic disturbances, and worsening of cognitive function for patients with Alzheimer's disease than for other patients and are only moderately effective in this population.

136. B: Seizures are rare in patients with multiple sclerosis, Parkinson's disease, and normal pressure hydrocephalus, but seizures do occur in stage 3 Alzheimer's disease.

137. A: The clinical triad described is highly suggestive of normal pressure hydrocephalus (NPH), a condition of unknown etiology in which excessive cerebrospinal fluid accumulates in the ventricles. The examination does not reveal papilledema, but ventricular enlargement is present on neuroimaging. Head trauma, subarachnoid hemorrhage, history of brain tumor, and central nervous system infection are all predisposing factors, but most cases occur independent of any of these factors. Surgical intervention is most likely to be beneficial when instituted early in the course of the disorder. The gait disturbance and urinary incontinence are most likely to be reversible; cognitive loss, once well established, is less likely to respond to shunting.

Donepezil is indicated for treatment of Alzheimer's disease. Carbidopa/levodopa is indicated for treatment of Parkinson's disease, in which gait disturbance can mimic NPH. Parkinson's disease, however, is more likely to be characterized by rigidity and tremor, which are absent in NPH. Dementia that is due to depression will respond to any intervention – behavioral or pharmacologic – that addresses the underlying depression.

138. D: Comment: While the clinical presentations of Alzheimer's Disease and multi-infarct dementia (MID) often overlap considerably, the distinguishing characteristic of MID, when present,

is the step-wise temporal progression, in contrast with the more continuous gradual decline of Alzheimer's Disease.

139. A: Obesity is the single greatest risk factor for the development of pseudotumor cerebri. Even a weight gain of 5% of body weight, falling well short of obesity, increases the risk. Weight loss is almost always a part of the comprehensive treatment plan forseudotumor cerebri. Cigarette smoking is probably not a risk factor. Various drugs, including oral contraceptives, lithium, tetracycline, and toxic doses of vitamin A, are all considered risk factors for developing pseudotumor, but the greatest risk factor is weight gain/obesity. Both steroid medication and abrupt discontinuation of steroid medication constitute risk factors for developing pseudotumor. Various underlying medical conditions may predispose to pseudotumor as well, including head injury, lupus, Lyme disease, and hypoparathyroidism. Weight gain/obesity still constitutes the greatest risk factor.

140. C: Herniation is an extremely uncommon complication of pseudotumor cerebri because the increased pressure is diffuse and builds gradually. Visual loss may occur because of buildup of pressure within the optic nerve sheath, and surgical fenestration of the sheath may be a necessary emergency surgical intervention to preserve eyesight for patients whose intracranial pressure does not decline with medical management.

141. D: Benign essential tremor involving the hands occurs preferentially when the hands are in use. Other parts of the body may also be involved with the tremor, including the head, which may bob from side to side or in the anterior-posterior sense. The tremor of Parkinson's disease occurs at rest. Cerebellar tremors typically occur most prominently at the end of a movement. Tremors due to toxic or metabolic abnormalities occur both at rest and with motion.

142. A: The clinical triad of tremor, rigidity, and bradykinesia in an older person is most likely to represent Parkinson's disease, which is the second most prevalent degenerative disease of older adults (after Alzheimer's disease). As the disease progresses, abnormal posture, impaired balance, and dementia often also ensue. Many patients develop difficulties with swallowing, including difficulty swallowing their own secretions. Some develop sleep abnormalities and autonomic instability. In the early stages of the disease, tremor may be the only symptom, but usually rigidity can be elicited on careful neurologic examination.

143. B: Although the exact cause of Parkinson's disease is unknown, it is clear that at a neurochemical level, the fundamental problem is depletion of dopaminergic neurons in brainstem and subcortical brain structures, including the substantia nigra, locus ceruleus, globus pallidus, and putamen. The dopamine cannot be replaced directly, because it is destroyed in the systemic circulation before it can reach the blood-brain barrier. Levodopa escapes this peripheral metabolism and crosses the blood-brain barrier. Levodopa is associated with multiple side effects, such as psychosis, anorexia, nausea, and vomiting, which can seriously limit its use in some patients.

144. C: Carbidopa is a competitive inhibitor of the enzyme dopa decarboxylase. Inhibiting this enzyme prevents levodopa from being converted to dopamine in the peripheral circulation before it can cross the blood-brain barrier. This helps to minimize adverse side-effects because it allows for lower serum concentrations of levodopa to achieve the desired levels within the brain. Elevating the serum concentration would be counter-productive in terms of side-effects. Entacapone prolongs the half-life of levodopa.

145. D: Many patients with Parkinson's disease develop difficulty with swallowing, putting them at risk for aspiration. These patients are already at risk for pneumonia because of their paucity of motor activity. The dietary modification most likely to be needed over time is to grind foods coarsely and serve them in small portions at frequent, supervised meals. Coarsely ground foods are easier for these patients to manipulate than soft foods and liquids. Some patients who take levodopa for symptom management will need to adjust the timing of their protein intake to accommodate their medication, because high levels of amino acids compete with levodopa for entry into the brain and reduce its effect. In this situation, it is best to have the main protein meal at a time of day when the patient can afford reduced physical activity. Patients with Parkinson's disease are at particular risk for falls and fractures, and they need protein, calcium, vitamin D, and weight-bearing exercise for bone integrity. It is the timing, not the amount, of protein intake that requires regulation.

146. A: Anticholinergic medications can be useful to treat tremor and to dry unmanageable secretions in patients with Parkinson's disease. This pharmacologic approach does not address rigidity or bradykinesia. Anticholinergic side-effects, such as constipation and urinary retention, limit the usefulness of this class of medications. There is no clear evidence that the anticholinergic drugs provide any neuroprotective effect in Parkinson's disease.

147. D: Comment: When a patient is about to undergo deep brain stimulation to treat symptoms of Parkinson's disease, dopaminergic medications are discontinued the night before surgery. This is to avoid medication-induced dyskinesias, which can distort intraoperative microelectrode recordings.

148. B: The pathologic mechanism of Wilson's disease is accumulation of zinc in various organs, including the brain, liver, kidneys, and eyes. Dietary zinc acetate competes with zinc for absorption and limits the amount of zinc absorbed from the intestinal tract. Zinc acetate may be used in asymptomatic patients who have come to diagnosis because of their family history; in these situations, the zinc acetate is intended to prevent zinc accumulation and its attendant end-organ damage. Zinc acetate therapy may also be used in Wilson's disease patients who have undergone chelation therapy to attempt to prevent recurrence of symptoms.

Vitamin D intake above 400IU/day is associated with lower incidence of multiple sclerosis and is frequently recommended for family members of individuals with multiple sclerosis. Folic acid deficiency is a risk factor for neural tube defects, such as spina bifida, and is recommended for pregnant women. Thiamine deficiency is a cause of Wernicke's encephalopathy.

149. D: Torticollis is the most common of the focal dystonias; blepharospasm is the second most common. Writer's cramp is less prevalent, although it is probably underdiagnosed. Torsion

dystonia is a rare generalized dystonia. Patients with dystonia have a defect in spinal reciprocal inhibition, the process by which antagonist muscles are made to relax when their paired agonists contract. There are also abnormalities of basal ganglia function and of sensory processing. Approximately half of the dystonias are inherited, mostly in an autosomal dominant manner; the remaining cases are either secondary (due to an underlying disease) or sporadic.

150. C: Attacks of hypokalemic periodic paralysis, which usually occurs on a hereditary (autosomal dominant) basis, can be precipitated by a high carbohydrate load, such as a meal of pasta. Alcohol and vigorous exercise precipitate attacks in some individuals. The underlying pathology consists of a range of abnormalities in ion channels in cell membranes.

151. B: Infants with Down syndrome master many of the same developmental tasks as other children, but it takes them longer to do so. The best outcomes are attainable with early, comprehensive, multidisciplinary intervention to provide abundant coordinated sensory, motor and cognitive experiences. In addition to the medical specialists required to address these children's spectrum of medical needs, the multidisciplinary team should include an audiologist, a physical therapist, an occupational therapist, and a speech therapist. These professionals can educate the parents and other family members to implement much of the child's treatment program independently.

Ketogenic diet can modestly reduce seizure frequency in patients with intractable epilepsy but has no role in the management of Down syndrome. A diet low in long-chain fatty acids, supplemented by Lorenzo's oil, can improve the course of adrenoleukodystrophy.

152. A: At autopsy, nearly all individuals with Down syndrome have the neuropathologic changes associated with Alzheimer's disease, namely neurofibrillary tangles and amyloid plaques. Not all of these individuals manifest actual cognitive decline, but by the age of 40, 11 – 24% of individuals with Down syndrome do develop actual dementia, and the percentage increases steeply with age, rising to 77% for individuals over the age of 60. Specialized cognitive instruments have been developed to assess cognitive decline in this population. The reason for the increased incidence of dementia in the Down syndrome population is not known. Limited data support the use of donepezil to treat dementia in patients with Down syndrome; results of a study of memantine in this population are pending.

Psychosis is less prevalent in individuals with Down syndrome than in the general population, although depression is common. Clinical anxiety disorders are also relatively uncommon in the Down syndrome population. While Down syndrome carries an increased risk of epilepsy over the general population, the risk is modest compared with the risk of dementia, with only 5 -10% of patients developing seizures over a lifetime.

153. C: Down syndrome is not an inherited disorder in the strict sense. Most cases, born to parents with no genetic abnormality, are caused by trisomy 21, which occurs due to errors in cell division during gametogenesis or early in the development of the embryo. When one parent has Down syndrome, however, the risk of Down syndrome or another developmental disorder is 35-50%. Women with Down syndrome develop sexually just as other women do and need comprehensive

sex education, not only for purposes of contraception, but also to avoid sexual abuse and sexually transmitted diseases.

154. D: Sleep apnea is extremely common in children and adults with Down syndrome because of their soft tissue abnormalities, including protruding tongue, receding chin, and thick neck. In some studies, nearly 100% of patients with Down syndrome had some degree of sleep apnea. Parents generally underestimate their children's sleep disturbance. Sleep apnea is a treatable cause of cognitive decline in any individual and a particularly important treatable cause of cognitive decline in individuals with Down syndrome. Epilepsy while slightly more common in individuals with Down syndrome than in the general population, is less prevalent than sleep apnea. Structural heart defects and rhythm disorders are also more common in the Down syndrome population, but less so than sleep apnea.

155. B: Babies with Down syndrome rarely need any particular special diet, but because they often have weakness of the facial muscles, protruding tongues, and other soft tissue abnormalities, they (and their mothers) need extra support with breast feeding and/or bottle feeding. Usually, it is enough to provide extra support for the neck and chin. Because of the shape of the nares, these babies may need gentle suctioning so that a stuffy nose does not interfere with oral intake. Auto immune disorders such as celiac disease and hypothyroidism are more common in the Down syndrome population than in the general population, but the most common nutritional support required is simple, practical assistance with normal intake of a normal diet.

156. C: Dependence and tolerance are physiologic responses to opioid medication that nearly every individual experiences to some extent, and patients should be educated to understand and expect these reactions. Dependence means that abrupt discontinuation of the medication will produce symptoms of withdrawal, which can be unpleasant and even life threatening. Because of this physiologic response, the patient should understand that when it is time to discontinue the medication, that process will be gradual and will require medical supervision. Tolerance means requiring increasing amounts of the medication over time in order to obtain the same level of analgesia. Since cross-tolerance among opioids is incomplete, one strategy for coping with tolerance is to simply change opioid analgesics if increasing the dose is not practical.

Addiction is a completely different phenomenon, which consists of using the medication in the absence of any clear medical need, continuing to use it in spite of harm to oneself, and committing antisocial acts to obtain it. In properly screened and supervised patients who are given long-acting or sustained-release opioids rather than short-acting preparations and who take their medication on a time-contingent rather than a pain-contingent regimen, addiction is very rare. In such patients, addiction is rare regardless of the diagnosis. Constipation, like other side effects of the opioid medications, is usually manageable, and usually recedes fairly quickly, as tolerance to the various opioid side effects builds rapidly in comparison to tolerance to the analgesic effect.

Patients embarking on opioid medication for long-term management of chronic pain need initial education and periodic educational reinforcement of these principles as do their family members and the various members of their medical team.

157. A: Dextromethorphan is an NMDA receptor antagonist. The development of opioid tolerance is mediated by central NMDA receptors.

158. C: Various pain conditions have characteristic diurnal signature patterns. Neuropathic pain, whether of peripheral or central origin, is usually most intense at night. Myofascial pain is usually bimodal with peak intensity in the morning and evening and partial relief in the middle of the day. Psychogenic pain – a diagnosis to be made only with great care – may lack any diurnal pattern.

159. D: Comment: Mononeuropathy simplex involves the distribution of a single peripheral nerve. Mononeuropathy multiplex involves several peripheral nerves in an asymmetric pattern scattered over distant segments of the body. Mononeuropathy multiplex may be produced by diabetes, but is distinct from diabetic peripheral polyneuropathy in clinical presentation, pathophysiology, and clinical course. When peripheral neuropathy is a remote effect of a malignant tumor (paraneoplastic syndrome), it is a pure sensory neuropathy.

160. C: Radial nerve compression or other injury can occur at almost any point along the course of the nerve, classically in the axilla through improper use of crutches or dangling the arm(s) over a chair ("Saturday night palsy"), at the level of the middle of the humerus through fractures, or over the distal forearm through repetitive use injury.

161. A: The inheritance of ALD is nearly always X-linked. Female carriers who have one abnormal allele on one X chromosome and one normal allele on the other X chromosome are generally asymptomatic, although some female carriers have a mild syndrome of progressive spasticity, weakness, and ataxia.

162. D: The adrenoleukodystrophies constitute a group of closely related genetic degenerative neurologic diseases caused by accumulation of very long chain fatty acids (VLCFA) due to lack of an enzyme that normally breaks these substances down. In the brain, the myelin sheath is damaged by excessive amounts of VLCFA. The adrenal cortex is also damaged by accumulations of VLCFA.

The glycogen storage diseases, of which Pompe Disease is an example, constitute a family of inherited disorders of glycogen metabolism, each caused by a different enzyme deficiency.

Alpha-glucosidase is the deficient enzyme in Pompe Disease.

Hexosaminidase is the enzyme missing in Tay - Sachs disease.

163. C: Women are three times more likely than men to develop carpal tunnel syndrome. Some of the increased incidence in women is related to fluid retention in the carpal tunnel during pregnancy, causing transient carpal tunnel syndrome that resolves spontaneously following delivery. In addition, several endocrine and auto-immune disorders that are more prevalent among women than men constitute risk factors for carpal tunnel syndrome. These include diabetes, hypothyroidism, rheumatoid arthritis, and celiac disease.

Parkinson's disease is more common in men than in women. Hormonal factors probably play a role – as yet undefined – as a longer total reproductive lifespan culminating in natural menopause has a modest protective effect. Adult-onset epilepsy is also slightly more common among men than among women. Alcoholism is more common among men than among women, although alcoholism in women is still likely under diagnosed.

164. B: The most common neurologic manifestation of HIV disease is peripheral neuropathy. Many different pathophysiologic mechanisms can be involved. Typically, HIV-related peripheral neuropathy is distal symmetrical polyneuropathy (DSPN) associated with advanced immunosuppression and/or toxicity of antiretroviral medications. Acute inflammatory demyelinating polyneuropathy (AIDP) generally occurs earlier in the course of HIV disease and may be the first manifestation of HIV infection. Mononeuropathy multiplex can be a primary neurologic manifestation of HIV disease as well. Individuals with HIV disease may also have peripheral neuropathy on the basis of intercurrent illnesses and toxic exposures that are related or unrelated to the HIV disease itself, such as various nutritional deficiencies and alcoholic peripheral neuropathy.

165. A: INH can cause pyridoxine deficiency, but the patient should be instructed to take pyridoxine supplements only as directed because this vitamin can be toxic at high concentrations. Replacement dosage for patients taking INH ranges from 10-50 mg/day. Children are generally less vulnerable than adults to INH-induced pyridoxine deficiency, but their risk increases with increasing INH dose and increasing duration of INH therapy, as well as with intercurrent nutritional deficiencies.

166. C: Teenage drivers with ADHD have four times more automobile accidents than other teenagers with comparable driving experience. Their accidents are more likely to cause injury, and teenagers with ADHD get three times as many speeding tickets as other teenagers. This does not mean that teenagers with ADHD should not drive, but it does highlight the need for excellent driver education, careful supervision, and extra attention to factors such as not driving while sleep-deprived and not engaging in distracting activities while driving.

Most children with ADHD continue to have symptoms during adolescence, although those symptoms may evolve. Some individuals with ADHD, especially those in whom hyperactivity is not prominent, may not be diagnosed until the teenage or adult years.

The decision to change or discontinue medication depends upon many factors. Because dose requirements change with growth, dose adjustment should be considered whenever the medication seems to have lost its effectiveness.

167. D: Restless leg syndrome can begin at any age, but the diagnosis is often missed during childhood when symptoms may be dismissed as "growing pains." Once established, however, symptoms of RLS often increase with age. Medications used for the treatment of Parkinson's Disease often help alleviate the symptoms of RLS, but people with RLS are no more likely than others in the general population to have Parkinson's Disease. Sometimes RLS appears during pregnancy; in these cases, the symptoms usually dissipate following delivery.

168. C: Patients with RLS are very heterogeneous in their responsiveness to various classes of medication. The most characteristic feature of their medication response is that no agent seems to be effective for very long. Therefore, the best strategy for pharmacologic management is usually cyclic deployment of the various classes of medication known to be effective, in a regimen individually tailored to each patient. Effective medications include anti-Parkinson's agents, opioids, benzodiazepines, muscle relaxants, and somenticonvulsants, particularly gabapentin. The tricyclic antidepressants often worsen symptoms of RLS, as do some anti-nausea drugs.

169. A: Although the statistical risk of progressive multifocal leukoencephalopathy (PML) is relatively small, this disease is progressive, debilitating, and almost always fatal. For this reason, natalizumab is reserved for patients whose multiple sclerosis has been unresponsive to standard treatment with interferons and glatiramer acetate and who have made a thoroughly considered an informed choice. There is also a 4% risk of allergic reaction, but these reactions almost always occur within 2 hours of initiating the infusion, so only short-term monitoring is required for this condition. Unlike the interferons, natalizumab has not been associated with any increased incidence of depression, and it does not cause flu-like side-effects or lipotrophy. Compliance is not a great concern because the drug is given by monthly intravenous infusion, and self-injection at home is not required.

170. D: Patients with depressed cellular immunity are at higher than average risk for development of PML. Among these patients, AIDS is the greatest risk factor, although antiretroviral treatments have contributed to a declining incidence of PML among individuals with HIV disease. Other conditions associated with immunosuppression also predispose to PML, including organ transplantation and leukemia, but AIDS remains the greatest risk factor. Multiple sclerosis is not directly associated with PML, but patients treated with natalizumab for MS have a 1 in 1000 risk of PML.

171. A: The existence of fibromyalgia as a legitimate medical disorder has been disputed because of the absence of an objective diagnostic test. Functional MRI examination,however, provides evidence both for hyperexcitability in central pain pathways of patients who meet the clinical criteria for fibromyalgia as well as reduced activity in descending central pain inhibitory pathways, lending credence to the understanding of fibromyalgia as a disorder of the central nervous system. The etiology remains unclear, although a novel virus has recently been reported in association with the disorder. It remains to be seen whether this virus will prove to have a causal relationship to fibromyalgia.

Because of their muscle tenderness, many fibromyalgia patients first present to rheumatologists who often manage the patients' medical care. Because of associated depression, these patients may also require psychiatric care, but fundamentally, fibromyalgia is neither a rheumatologic nor a psychiatric disorder. As with any disorder, there are some individuals who exploit the symptoms of fibromyalgia for non-medical gain, but fibromyalgia is not a form of malingering.

172. D: During an attack, activities such as reading and watching television and stimuli such as bright lights and loud noises can exacerbate the vertigo. Lying down and resting is the best approach.

173. D: Because vertigo associated with Ménière's Disease can lead to falls or injury while driving, operating machinery, or performing any task that involves changes in position, it is extremely important to make the individualized lifestyle changes necessary for safety. The unpleasantness of the symptoms of the disease itself, coupled with restricted lifestyle, predisposes patients to depression.

174. B: The expectations of the physician and patient should be explicitly documented as a permanent part of the medical record, and copies should be sent to relevant members of the medical team, including the pharmacist and other physicians. This document should specify that the patient will not seek or receive prescriptions for controlled substances from any other provider, will fill prescriptions at the same pharmacy every month, will not seek new prescriptions prematurely, and will cooperate with random urine and/or blood tests for opioid levels. Further, the document should state that failure to meet these obligations will result in discontinuation of the professional relationship.

Short-acting opioids that the patient may have been taking on a pain-contingent basis are discontinued SIMULTANEOUSLY with initiating a time-contingent regimen of sustained-release opioid medication. Dextromethorphan is often added to chronic opioid regimens to attempt to prevent the development of tolerance. In this situation, the addition of dextromethorphan is delayed until a week or more after initiation of the new regimen in order to allow tolerance to the unwanted side-effects to develop. Tolerance to side-effects, such as nausea, constipation, and respiratory suppression develops rapidly and is desirable; tolerance to analgesia develops more slowly. Psychological evaluation is often helpful, and some practitioners require it in every case while others obtain psychological evaluation in selected cases only.

175. C: Although many patients with low back pain attributed to degenerative disc disease fear increasing pain with time, the opposite is more often the case. This is probably because the nucleus pulposus eventually becomes depleted of the inflammatory proteins responsible for much of the pain, and the annulus fibrosus stiffens, reducing the micro-motion that likely contributes to discogenic pain. While other causes of low back pain increase with age, pain due to degenerative disc disease actually decreases with age. Thus, it is not justified to offer surgery to a symptomatic younger person simply as a strategy to avoid increased pain or the need for surgery in later years.

176. B: Sitting is often the most painful position for a patient with degenerative lumbar disc disease because the discs are maximally loaded (three times more than in the standing position) with the patient seated. Walking, and even running, may offer temporary pain relief. Lateral rotation generally does not affect the pain, and a report of increased pain with lateral rotation should arouse suspicion of malingering. Lying down usually provides a measure of relief.

177. B: In children, spondylolisthesis is most often congenital. This is dysplastic spondylolisthesis, and is caused by abnormal formation of a facet, which allows the vertebral body to slide anteriorly. Traumatic spondylolisthesis can occur at any age, especially in individuals who engage in contact sports or activities that require repetitive hyperextension. Degenerative (arthritic) spondylolisthesis is a condition of older adults.

178. C: Multiple system atrophy is a syndrome of unknown etiology characterized by motor symptoms similar to those of Parkinson's disease, along with a variety of autonomic disturbances, especially orthostatic hypotension. As the disease progresses, however, central respiratory drive fails, and patients often die in their sleep because they simply fail to breathe. These patients often have swallowing problems, and aspiration is a risk, but this risk is manageable, and patients with multiple system atrophy typically do not die either of malnutrition or aspiration.

179. A: Among the many autonomic disturbances that can occur in individuals with multiple system atrophy, hyperthermia with heat stroke is among the most potentially lethal. When these patients develop hyperthermia, it is because they cannot sweat.

180. D: Obesity, while a risk factor for a number of adverse health outcomes, is actually a protective factor for vertebral fracture while low body weight, even in the absence of osteoporosis, is an independent risk factor for vertebral fracture.

181. C: Pain caused by lumbar spinal stenosis generally abates somewhat with bending forward. Since this is the posture assumed when walking uphill, walking uphill is associated with less pain than walking downhill. This is the opposite of vascular claudication, which is more severe walking uphill than downhill because of the increased muscular work involved. While pain due to degenerative lumbar disc disease is worse when sitting than when standing because of the increased load on the disc(s), the pain of lumbar spinal stenosis is worse when standing and partially or even completely relieved by sitting.

182. A: The primary risk factor for spinal stenosis is age. Other risk factors come into play in a minority of cases. These include skeletal fluorosis, Paget disease of the spine, congenital malformations, and achondroplasia, which is associated with an abnormally narrow spinal canal.

183. D: Even in neonates with open fontanelles, untreated hydrocephalus generally has a poor outcome, especially if associated with central nervous system infection or tumor. The fatality rate is 50-60%, and among survivors, intellectual and other neurological deficits are common. Treatment may consist of shunting, surgically removing any existing blockage, or damaging the cells of the choroid plexus that manufacture cerebrospinal fluid.

184. B: An advance directive is a document that sets forth an individual's wishes concerning his health care in the event that he becomes unable to make such decisions for himself. A living will is a restricted type of advance directive that confines its instructions to end of-life care. A durable power of attorney for health care names a specific individual and authorizes that person to make health care decisions on the individual's behalf if he becomes unable to make such decisions for himself. The individual so designated is the health care proxy (health care agent.)

185. C: The varicella-zoster vaccine (Zostavax) is a live attenuated virus that is recommended for all adults over age 60 who have had chickenpox and who have no compromise of their immune system, whether they have had an episode of zoster or not. This live-virus vaccine is not recommended for individuals with conditions that compromise the immune system, such as AIDS, cancer chemotherapy, bone marrow or lymphatic cancer, or treatment with steroids.

186. At: The triptan medications are very effective for aborting established migraine attacks and help to reduce not only pain but also associated symptoms such as nausea, vomiting, and photosensitivity. They should not be taken, however, by individuals with hypertension, history of coronary heart disease, or significant risk factors for heart attack or stroke.

187. B: Multiple studies show consistently better cognitive function over time in multiple sclerosis (MS) patients who begin disease modifying therapy soon after diagnosis. Results are consistent for interferon and glatiramer acetate therapy with results influenced more by timing of intervention than by the choice of disease-modifying agent. Results with natalizumab are particularly striking, not only for prevention of long-term cognitive decline, but also for reversal of existing cognitive impairments and rapidity of onset of the effect. It is thought that most of the benefit conferred by disease-modifying agents is attributable to prevention of the inflammatory processes that dominate the early pathophysiology of MS and lead to the later, more refractory, degenerative pathophysiologic phases of MS.

There is some evidence to suggest that donepezil has a modest benefit in reducing long-term cognitive decline in patients with MS. Conceptually, it is more appealing to address cognitive decline in MS proactively with disease-modifying strategies than to address the issue symptomatically after the fact with anticholinesterase inhibitors.

There is no evidence to support the use of memantine to treat MS-related cognitive impairment. In one study, MS patients treated with memantine scored worse than controls on certain measurements of cognitive function.

Studies show modest benefit with l-amphetamine on certain secondary measures of cognitive function in patients with MS.

It is worth noting that in normal controls, higher serum levels of 25-hydroxyvitamin D are associated with better performance on tests of cognitive function. Vitamin D is currently being explored for its potential to delay cognitive decline and/or promote cognitive improvement in patients with MS.

188. D: Subcutaneously administered disease-modifying agents are associated with injection site reactions ranging from mild erythema to lipotrophy. Lesions are associated with a range of levels of pain, redness induration, tissue destruction, and residual scarring. Unlike other side effects of disease-modifying therapy, injection site reactions tend to be persistent over time and constitute a challenge for long-term compliance with treatment. Injection into the subcutaneous space allows the agent to encounter the body's full arsenal of immune responsiveness while injection into the more immunologically isolated skeletal muscle avoids such reactivity.

Various strategies to minimize injection site reactions can be helpful for some patients. These include pretreatment with oral anti-inflammatory medication and topical ice, and initiating therapy with a low dose to be gradually escalated. Good injection technique is essential, and automated injection devices help some patients.

189. B: The patient's right to self-determination takes precedence. Beneficence, the mandate to act in the best interest of the patient, is informed by the patient's own sense of what is actually good for him. Dignity is also understood to conform to the patient's own sense of what is dignified and respectful, even if family members and health professionals have conflicting views of what constitutes dignity. Justice, meaning a fair distribution of resources, is not in question in this case, regardless of the ultimate decision.

190. D: Extreme caution is necessary in determining brain death. In particular, it should be noted that various medications, including barbiturates, opioids, benzodiazepines, tricyclic antidepressants, anticonvulsants, aminoglycosides, and others can interfere with tests of various brainstem functions. In addition, brain death should not be declared definitively in the absence of a catastrophic event that can reasonably account for it.

191. D: Zostavax is a live attenuated virus vaccine indicated for prevention of shingles in immunocompetent adults over age 60. Shingles is caused by reactivation of dormant varicella-zoster virus. The syndrome of shingles is also called herpes zoster, but it is not caused by the herpes simplex virus. Because Zostavax is a live attenuated virus, it is possible to transmit the virus from a recently vaccinated individual to a vulnerable host. Recently vaccinated individuals should avoid close contact with immunosuppressed persons and pregnant women. In the United States, less than 10% of the population for whom this vaccine is intended has actually been vaccinated.

192. C: Of the conditions listed above, only postherpetic neuralgia (PHN) has a significant sympathetically maintained component. Sympathetic blockade, if provided early in the course of shingles, can shorten the duration of the cutaneous outbreak and pain and reduce the likelihood of developing PHN. For established PHN, sympathetic blockade can also shorten the duration of the syndrome. Earlier intervention carries the greatest chance for benefit.

Since most cases of shingles resolve without long-lasting pain, the decision to intervene with an invasive procedure should be carefully considered. In general, the risk of postherpetic neuralgia increases significantly with age. The site of the cutaneous eruption does not influence the likelihood of postherpetic neuralgia, but certain sites are associated with particularly impaired quality of life if PHN does ensue. Patients with involvement of the ophthalmic division of the trigeminal nerve are particularly debilitated if PHN ensues.

193. B: A spinal headache is characterized by continuous, dull ache, particularly severe through the mid-face. The headache is exacerbated by sitting or standing and is substantially, or even completely, relieved by lying flat. The pain may be accompanied by nausea. The most common cause, even with meticulous technique and narrow-gauge needles, is lumbar puncture performed either for diagnostic purposes or for spinal anesthesia. Sometimes, however, a condition of spontaneous intracranial hypotension arises in the absence of any instrumentation of the dura. The headache is the same as classic spinal headache and may be accompanied by nausea, vertigo, radicular pain in the upper extremities, or intermittent hearing loss. The cause is spontaneous dural leak of CSF; it is not always clear what produces the leak, although sometimes connective tissue disorders are implicated. Opening pressure on diagnostic lumbar puncture may be low or normal, and a normal opening pressure does not exclude spontaneous intracranial hypotension. CT

myelogram offers the best opportunity for diagnosis and is likely to reveal leakage of CSF at cervical and/or thoracic nerve root sleeves as well as dural diverticula at the root sleeves.

Whether due to lumbar puncture or to spontaneous intracranial hypotension, spinal headache usually responds to placement of a blood patch. Sometimes more than one patch is required, and sometimes surgical repair of the torn root sleeves is required to treat spontaneous intracranial hypotension.

194. A: Huntington's disease most typically presents with cognitive symptoms in early middle age. Patients whose symptoms begin earlier often have a more rapidly debilitating course, and they are more likely to present with motor signs such as rigidity, bradykinesia, and tremor before displaying signs of cognitive decline. Patients whose symptoms begin earlier in life are also at greater risk of seizures.

195. C: Huntington's disease is caused by a single gene with autosomal dominance and complete penetrance. Thus with each mating involving one parent with Huntington's disease, there is a 50% chance of the defective allele being inherited. Because environmental factors do not contribute to the disorder, a person who inherits the allele for Huntington's disease is certain to develop the disease if he lives until middle age. In rare instances, Huntington's disease arises through a spontaneous mutation. Because the disease does not present clinically until a person is well into the adult reproductive years, genetic diagnosis is complicated by a variety of psychological and ethical factors.

196. B: Ideally, antibiotic treatment for neurosyphilis at any stage and with any combination of neurologic symptoms should be accomplished with intravenous aqueous crystalline Penicillin G every four hours for 10-14 days. This may or may not be followed by 3 weekly doses of benzathine Penicillin G to address the possibility of slowly reproducing organisms that are not eradicated by the initial regimen. In the event of allergy to Penicillin, a 14-day course of daily intramuscular ceftriaxone is acceptable.

The Jarisch-Herxheimer reaction is not a contraindication to antibiotic treatment for syphilis at any stage. In fact, Jarisch-Herxheimer reaction is most common in treatment of secondary syphilis and least common in treatment of late syphilis. The reaction, if it occurs, is usually mild and confined to the first dose of antibiotic and can be attenuated by pretreatment with acetaminophen or prednisone. While most syphilis occurs in HIV-infected individuals, there is no need to treat every syphilis patient for HIV, since excellent diagnostic tools for HIV infection are available, and HAART entails an intensive and costly regimen and carries risks for significant side effects.

197. D: In many hospitals, anesthesiologists refuse to provide epidural obstetric anesthesia to mothers with multiple sclerosis. The idea that epidural anesthesia can precipitate an exacerbation of MS, however, is entirely unsupported by clinical research. In some communities, the policy to withhold epidural anesthesia is based on fear of legal action if the woman does indeed have an exacerbation of her MS. Since the post-partum period is a time of heightened risk of exacerbation, the concern is understandable, but it is the sudden change in hormonal environment, not the

epidural injection or anesthetic agent, that is responsible for the high rate of exacerbations in the weeks following childbirth.

A newborn whose mother has multiple sclerosis is at no greater risk of medical complications than any other newborn. There should be no confusion with neonatal myasthenia gravis.

198. A: Subacute sclerosing panencephalitis is a rare neurologic complication of measles infection. Onset is years (rarely months) after a bout of measles that has apparently resolved. The condition usually presents with subtle cognitive decline and personality change and progresses to frank dementia accompanied by spasticity, ataxia, myoclonus, and seizures. The condition is nearly always fatal, although if treatment with varying combinations of isoprinosine and interferon alpha is instituted in the early stages and continued indefinitely, the patient may survive with relative neurologic stability. The disease is thought to be caused by a mutation in the measles virus and is nearly 100% preventable with vaccination.

199. C: Reye's syndrome is a syndrome of unknown etiology consisting of encephalopathy and hepatocellular damage. It usually occurs a week or more following recovery from a febrile illness, especially chickenpox or influenza, during which the patient has been treated with aspirin or other salicylates. Children between the ages of 4 and 12 years are most at risk. Symptoms include altered personality and behavior, which may progress to delirium, seizures and coma along with vomiting and liver dysfunction characterized by elevated hepatocellular enzyme levels and elevated blood ammonia level. There is no specific treatment, but aggressive supportive care is required. Mortality is as high as 40% in some series. The only modifiable risk factor is exposure to salicylates.

200. D: The risk factor most strongly linked to development of Guillain-Barré syndrome is recent bacterial or viral illness. The exact pathophysiologic mechanism is not known, but the evidence supports an autoimmune process in which the myelin of peripheral nerves is damaged. The antecedent infection that most commonly precedes GBS is Campylobacter jejuni. Influenza is a notorious, but actually less common antecedent illness. Although peripheral myelin is the tissue targeted for damage in GBS, there is no evidence that patients who develop GBS following an infectious illness have any inherent abnormality of myelin.

During the influenza immunization campaign of 1976, approximately 500 cases of GBS were reported among those who received the vaccine, and some 25 cases proved fatal. This cluster of cases has been attributed to the vaccine itself, but no influenza vaccine before or since has been linked to an outbreak of GBS beyond the normal background incidence.

201. A: Locked-in syndrome consists of total inability to speak or move other than vertical eye movements and blinking, without any impairment of consciousness or cognition. Usually, it is caused by damage to the central pons. The pathologic process can be trauma, stroke, tumor, demyelination, or metabolic injury. A similar syndrome can occasionally be produced by Guillain-Barré syndrome, although on a completely different neuroanatomic basis. A simple system of communication using eye blinking and the preserved vertical eye movements suffices as a first step in bedside communication until sophisticated technologies can be brought to bear to facilitate communication. Whatever code is established, it should be clearly

posted for all to see at the head of the patient's bed. Everyone involved in the patient's care should be reminded that the patient has full cognitive function and can comprehend everything that he would normally have comprehended prior to this neurologic disaster.

202. C: The goal is to stop the seizures as quickly as possible. The benzodiazepines are preferred for their rapid onset of action, and lorazepam is the drug of choice because of its long duration of action. Midazolam can be given intramuscularly if intravenous access cannot be established. If seizures continue, then the patient can be loaded with fosphenytoin or phenytoin if serum levels are subtherapeutic. Phenobarbital is also effective for managing status epilepticus but has the disadvantage of sedation and respiratory suppression.

203. B: The most serious complication of idiopathic intracranial hypertension is visual loss due to optic nerve injury. The onset of visual loss may be insidious, and acuity testing alone is not sufficiently sensitive monitoring. During treatment for idiopathic intracranial hypertension, a patient requires regular formal visual field examination. Visual loss related to idiopathic intracranial hypertension can be permanent, so immediate intervention is required if vision is compromised. The most direct approach is optic nerve sheath fenestration. Measures such as therapeutic lumbar puncture or shunting that lower intracranial pressure may also be effective.

204. B: Attacks of daytime sleepiness associated with narcolepsy can occur when the patient is under stimulated (bored) or when he is engaged in complex activity such as driving. Sometimes there is a brief warning, but often there is none at all, and individuals with inadequately treated narcolepsy have a high rate of automobile collisions and fatalities.

Although the sleep attack in narcolepsy is irresistible, a person experiencing such an attack can be roused just as from normal sleep. At the end of the episode, the patient usually awakens feeling refreshed, but the feeling may not last, and another attack may ensue shortly.

The underlying abnormality of sleep architecture in narcolepsy is intrusion of REM sleep, including its associated motor paralysis into waking life. Hence, there is dreaming during the episodes of daytime sleep.

205. C: Hyperthermia increases metabolic needs of all tissues, including the brain. Hyperthermia following acute stroke accelerates pathologic changes in the affected brain tissue and promotes extension of the area of damage. Elevated temperatures should be treated promptly with antipyretics for the sake of protecting the brain, and the underlying cause should be found and treated as well if possible.

206. D: Bleeding is the most common complication of rt-PA for any indication. Following rt-PA for ischemic stroke, the risk of intracerebral bleeding is added to the risks of peripheral bleeding. Even if the patient is going to need anticoagulation ultimately, no anticoagulation is indicated during the first 24 hours following administration of rt-PA for ischemic stroke. During this time, the patient has to be examined regularly for any signs of peripheral bleeding. Oral hygiene is limited t mouthwashes and soft sponges, and the patient should not shave. Peripheral IV sites and any pre-existing sores or wounds are inspected for evidence of bleeding. If anticoagulation is contemplated

after the first 24 hours, a brain CT is required first to rule out any unsuspected intracranial bleeding.

207. A: Alzheimer's disease is a terminal disease. Educating families to this reality is important because unlike patients with other terminal diseases, many patients with Alzheimer's disease fail to receive appropriate end-of-life care. For example, patients dying with Alzheimer's disease are far less likely than patients dying of cancer to be referred for hospice care. Likewise, patients with Alzheimer's disease are more likely than others to undergo invasive procedures in the last months of life. Both situations are driven by unrealistic expectations on the part of families. The fact that Alzheimer's disease is a terminal disease needs to be repeated multiple times.

208. C: Only riluzole is associated with extended survival time and extended time to tracheostomy in patients with ALS. High-dose vitamin E is not recommended because no benefit is established; low-dose vitamin E is insufficiently studied. High-dose creatine has also been evaluated and found to be of no demonstrable benefit in ALS. Riluzole does show modest benefit in extending survival and time to tracheostomy. The drug is associated with quite frequent side effects, such as nausea, sedation, dizziness, and transient elevation of transaminases. Since ALS remains a terminal disease, considerations of quality of life come into play in deciding whether to continue riluzole in the face of side effects.

209. D: Symptoms of vascular dementia usually present in step-wise fashion. Periods of stability are punctuated by episodes of decline. This clinical pattern correlates with the presumed pathology, which consists of multiple small infarcts – usually subcortical and not resulting in obvious deficits outside the cognitive realm. The other dementias listed are more likely to progress in a gradual, continuous manner. It should be noted that the dementia associated with depression is a true dementia, and depression is among the treatable causes of dementia.

210. B: Symptoms of vascular dementia usually present in step-wise fashion. Periods of stability are punctuated by episodes of decline. This clinical pattern correlates with the presumed pathology, which consists of multiple small infarcts – usually subcortical and not resulting in obvious deficits outside the cognitive realm. The other dementias listed are more likely to progress in a gradual, continuous manner. It should be noted that the dementia associated with depression is a true dementia, and depression is among the treatable causes of dementia.

211. D: Some patients with obstructive sleep apnea may require CPAP, some may require surgery, and some may require weight loss, but these measures alone are typically not successful in the absence of comprehensive lifestyle changes that include a regular schedule and routine for sleep, correct sleep position, and avoidance of cigarettes and alcohol.

212. A: Lactulose is indicated for its ability to lower the intestinal burden of ammonia-producing bacteria as well as clearing blood from the intestines in the event of GI bleed. Neomycin and rifaximin may also be used for the same purpose in the context of hepatic encephalopathy. Any medications that rely on hepatic function for clearance are contraindicated unless absolutely necessary for life-saving purposes. If such medications are required, then dose size and dose

interval have to be corrected to take into account the impaired hepatic function. Likewise, medications that are likely to contribute to sedation are contraindicated. While seizures can occur late in the course of hepatic encephalopathy, most patients with hepatic encephalopathy do not experience seizures, and anticonvulsant medication does not need to be added prophylactically, especially since most anticonvulsants are metabolized via the liver and can contribute to sedation when first initiated.

213. D: This patient is experiencing delirium superimposed on her early Alzheimer's disease. Delirium is extremely common in elderly hospitalized patients. Although delirium usually resolves within a week, it often takes much longer for the patient to fully return to baseline mental status. Delirium is also a poor prognostic sign as 25% or more of individuals who develop dementia during a hospital stay die in hospital, and 25% or more die within the year. Delirium may also mark the onset of dementia. Delirium may be caused simply by disruption of familiar routines and separation from familiar surroundings. Both at home and in hospital, medications, drug interactions, and withdrawal from medications are very frequently the cause of delirium, and unless the patient's agitated behavior puts him or others at risk, it is best to avoid adding yet more medication to the regimen to control the disruptive behaviors.

Regardless of the underlying cause or causes, the patient's environment should be normalized to the extent possible. The room should have natural daylight during the day, with a view of the outdoors and should be quiet and dark at night. Family members or a sitter should be present for as much of the time as is comfortable for the patient, and the patient should be given verbal and non-verbal orientation frequently. Music and physical touch are also helpful.

214. C: Neuromyelitis optica (Devic's disease) is a central nervous system demyelinating disorder distinct from and much less common than multiple sclerosis. Attacks of unilateral or bilateral optic neuritis and/or myelitis typically have a devastatingly disabling effect, and treatments that are effective for multiple sclerosis are generally not effective, although some patients do respond to immunosuppression with glucocorticoids, azathioprine, cyclophosphamide, or mycophenolate.

The most specific laboratory marker for neuromyelitis optica is serum NMO antibody. The CSF profile usually shows mild lymphocytic pleocytosis and elevated protein, but no oligoclonal bands.

215. A: The classic triad of fever, focal neurologic abnormalities, and increased intracranial pressure is often incomplete in the early stages of brain abscess. Untreated, most brain abscesses will eventually bloom into this triad of findings, progressing, often rapidly, to fatality in the absence of intervention. Surgery is usually required in addition to systemic antibiotics, because antibiotics do not penetrate the abscess very well. In addition, it is essential to find and treat the underlying cause that gave rise to the abscess in the first place. The emphasis should be on finding and treating sources of infective emboli, such as endocarditis, sources of right-to-left shunts such as heart defects, or conditions causing immunosuppression.

216. B: Craniopharyngiomas suprasellar tumors that arise from embryonic remnants of the craniopharyngeal duct or Rathke's cleft. Because of their location, they mimic pituitary adenomas in neurologic and endocrine presentation. They are typically cystic, containing viscous material that

has been compared to motor oil. While these tumors are histologically benign, they may recur following resection, probably because complete resection is not always possible. Complete surgical resection is the preferred approach whenever possible; when not possible, surgery may be followed by radiation therapy, but craniopharyngiomas are not responsive to chemotherapy.

217. C: Both central and obstructive sleep apnea are very common among patients with post-polio syndrome, although disordered breathing during sleep is often overlooked as a significant contributing factor in the fatigue these patients typically experience. Sleep apnea occurs as a feature of post-polio syndrome both in patients who have had bulbar poliomyelitis and in patients who have had spinal poliomyelitis as the initial infection. Treatment of the sleep disorder has to be individualized.

Post-polio syndrome, which follows acute poliomyelitis infection by decades, is most likely to occur in patients who have made a good recovery from the initial infection. This probably reflects the nature of the process of recovery from polio in which surviving anterior horn cells take over the function of destroyed motor neurons, innervating larger motor units. With aging, anterior horn cells are normally lost, and with the loss of each anterior horn cell, a larger than normal motor unit loses function. The mechanism of post-polio syndrome is probably not auto-immune in nature, and the diagnosis does not rely on immune markers or evidence of abnormal immune activity in the blood or in the cerebrospinal fluid. On EMG examination, post-polio patients exhibit evidence of anterior horn cell disease, namely increased amplitude and duration or motor action potentials and increased percentage of polyphasic potentials.

218. D: Pure mental neuropathy consists of unilateral numbness on the chin in the distribution of the mental nerve, which is a branch of the mandibular division of the trigeminal nerve. In the vast majority of cases, this syndrome represents metastatic cancer. Some previously unsuspected malignancies present with mental neuropathy; more commonly, recurrent tumor with metastatic spread announces itself in this fashion.

219. B: Hypothermia drives extracellular potassium into the cells, leading to serum hypokalemia. When the patient is rewarmed, potassium shifts back to the extracellular fluid. It may be necessary to replace serum potassium during hypothermia, but this should be done cautiously, knowing that hyperkalemia may ensue as the patient is rewarmed. During rewarming, the patient's IV fluids should not contain potassium, and potassium-wasting agents may be required.

220. D: The incidence of Bell's palsy is significantly higher among patients with diabetes than in any other disease grouping, so a patient with Bell's palsy should always be evaluated for the possibility of underlying diabetes. This is especially important, since prednisolone, previously considered a somewhat controversial treatment, has recently been shown to be significantly more effective than placebo in outcome of Bell's palsy if initiated within 72 hours of onset of symptoms. Antivirals, by contrast, have not been demonstrated to be effective in improving outcomes for patients with Bell's palsy.

Young patients presenting with trigeminal neuralgia should be evaluated for possible multiple sclerosis. In general, the neurologic examination alone is sufficient to differentiate Bell's palsy from stroke. Patients with unilateral pure mental neuropathy should be aggressively evaluated for metastatic malignancy.

Secret Key #1 - Time is Your Greatest Enemy

Pace Yourself

Wear a watch. At the beginning of the test, check the time (or start a chronometer on your watch to count the minutes), and check the time after every few questions to make sure you are "on schedule."

If you are forced to speed up, do it efficiently. Usually one or more answer choices can be eliminated without too much difficulty. Above all, don't panic. Don't speed up and just begin guessing at random choices. By pacing yourself, and continually monitoring your progress against your watch, you will always know exactly how far ahead or behind you are with your available time. If you find that you are one minute behind on the test, don't skip one question without spending any time on it, just to catch back up. Take 15 fewer seconds on the next four questions, and after four questions you'll have caught back up. Once you catch back up, you can continue working each problem at your normal pace.

Furthermore, don't dwell on the problems that you were rushed on. If a problem was taking up too much time and you made a hurried guess, it must be difficult. The difficult questions are the ones you are most likely to miss anyway, so it isn't a big loss. It is better to end with more time than you need than to run out of time.

Lastly, sometimes it is beneficial to slow down if you are constantly getting ahead of time. You are always more likely to catch a careless mistake by working more slowly than quickly, and among very high-scoring test takers (those who are likely to have lots of time left over), careless errors affect the score more than mastery of material.

Secret Key #2 - Guessing is not Guesswork

You probably know that guessing is a good idea - unlike other standardized tests, there is no penalty for getting a wrong answer. Even if you have no idea about a question, you still have a 20-25% chance of getting it right.

Most test takers do not understand the impact that proper guessing can have on their score. Unless you score extremely high, guessing will significantly contribute to your final score.

Monkeys Take the Test

What most test takers don't realize is that to insure that 20-25% chance, you have to guess randomly. If you put 20 monkeys in a room to take this test, assuming they answered once per question and behaved themselves, on average they would get 20-25% of the questions correct. Put 20 test takers in the room, and the average will be much lower among guessed questions. Why?

1. The test writers intentionally writes deceptive answer choices that "look" right. A test taker has no idea about a question, so picks the "best looking" answer, which is often wrong. The monkey has no idea what looks good and what doesn't, so will consistently be lucky about 20-25% of the time.

2. Test takers will eliminate answer choices from the guessing pool based on a hunch or intuition. Simple but correct answers often get excluded, leaving a 0% chance of being correct. The monkey has no clue, and often gets lucky with the best choice.

This is why the process of elimination endorsed by most test courses is flawed and detrimental to your performance- test takers don't guess, they make an ignorant stab in the dark that is usually worse than random.

$5 Challenge

Let me introduce one of the most valuable ideas of this course- the $5 challenge:

You only mark your "best guess" if you are willing to bet $5 on it.
You only eliminate choices from guessing if you are willing to bet $5 on it.

Why $5? Five dollars is an amount of money that is small yet not insignificant, and can really add up fast (20 questions could cost you $100). Likewise, each answer choice on one question of the test will have a small impact on your overall score, but it can really add up to a lot of points in the end.

The process of elimination IS valuable. The following shows your chance of guessing it right:

If you eliminate wrong answer choices until only this many remain:	1	2	3
Chance of getting it correct:	100%	50%	33%

However, if you accidentally eliminate the right answer or go on a hunch for an incorrect answer, your chances drop dramatically: to 0%. By guessing among all the answer choices, you are GUARANTEED to have a shot at the right answer.

That's why the $5 test is so valuable- if you give up the advantage and safety of a pure guess, it had better be worth the risk.

What we still haven't covered is how to be sure that whatever guess you make is truly random. Here's the easiest way:

Always pick the first answer choice among those remaining.

Such a technique means that you have decided, **before you see a single test question**, exactly how you are going to guess- and since the order of choices tells you nothing about which one is correct, this guessing technique is perfectly random.

This section is not meant to scare you away from making educated guesses or eliminating choices- you just need to define when a choice is worth eliminating. The $5 test, along with a pre-defined random guessing strategy, is the best way to make sure you reap all of the benefits of guessing.

Secret Key #3 - Practice Smarter, Not Harder

Many test takers delay the test preparation process because they dread the awful amounts of practice time they think necessary to succeed on the test. We have refined an effective method that will take you only a fraction of the time.

There are a number of "obstacles" in your way to succeed. Among these are answering questions, finishing in time, and mastering test-taking strategies. All must be executed on the day of the test at peak performance, or your score will suffer. The test is a mental marathon that has a large impact on your future.

Just like a marathon runner, it is important to work your way up to the full challenge. So first you just worry about questions, and then time, and finally strategy:

Success Strategy

1. Find a good source for practice tests.
2. If you are willing to make a larger time investment, consider using more than one study guide- often the different approaches of multiple authors will help you "get" difficult concepts.
3. Take a practice test with no time constraints, with all study helps "open book." Take your time with questions and focus on applying strategies.
4. Take a practice test with time constraints, with all guides "open book."
5. Take a final practice test with no open material and time limits

If you have time to take more practice tests, just repeat step 5. By gradually exposing yourself to the full rigors of the test environment, you will condition your mind to the stress of test day and maximize your success.

Secret Key #4 - **Prepare, Don't Procrastinate**

Let me state an obvious fact: if you take the test three times, you will get three different scores.

This is due to the way you feel on test day, the level of preparedness you have, and, despite the test writers' claims to the contrary, some tests WILL be easier for you than others.

Since your future depends so much on your score, you should maximize your chances of success. In order to maximize the likelihood of success, you've got to prepare in advance. This means taking practice tests and spending time learning the information and test taking strategies you will need to succeed.

Never take the test as a "practice" test, expecting that you can just take it again if you need to. Feel free to take sample tests on your own, but when you go to take the official test, be prepared, be focused, and do your best the first time!

Secret Key #5 - Test Yourself

Everyone knows that time is money. There is no need to spend too much of your time or too little of your time preparing for the test. You should only spend as much of your precious time preparing as is necessary for you to get the score you need.

Once you have taken a practice test under real conditions of time constraints, then you will know if you are ready for the test or not.

If you have scored extremely high the first time that you take the practice test, then there is not much point in spending countless hours studying. You are already there.

Benchmark your abilities by retaking practice tests and seeing how much you have improved. Once you score high enough to guarantee success, then you are ready.

If you have scored well below where you need, then knuckle down and begin studying in earnest. Check your improvement regularly through the use of practice tests under real conditions. Above all, don't worry, panic, or give up. The key is perseverance!

Then, when you go to take the test, remain confident and remember how well you did on the practice tests. If you can score high enough on a practice test, then you can do the same on the real thing.

General Strategies

The most important thing you can do is to ignore your fears and jump into the test immediately- do not be overwhelmed by any strange-sounding terms. You have to jump into the test like jumping into a pool- all at once is the easiest way.

Make Predictions

As you read and understand the question, try to guess what the answer will be. Remember that several of the answer choices are wrong, and once you begin reading them, your mind will immediately become cluttered with answer choices designed to throw you off. Your mind is typically the most focused immediately after you have read the question and digested its contents. If you can, try to predict what the correct answer will be. You may be surprised at what you can predict.

Quickly scan the choices and see if your prediction is in the listed answer choices. If it is, then you can be quite confident that you have the right answer. It still won't hurt to check the other answer choices, but most of the time, you've got it!

Answer the Question

It may seem obvious to only pick answer choices that answer the question, but the test writers can create some excellent answer choices that are wrong. Don't pick an answer just because it sounds right, or you believe it to be true. It MUST answer the question. Once you've made your selection, always go back and check it against the question and make sure that you didn't misread the question, and the answer choice does answer the question posed.

Benchmark

After you read the first answer choice, decide if you think it sounds correct or not. If it doesn't, move on to the next answer choice. If it does, mentally mark that answer choice. This doesn't mean that you've definitely selected it as your answer choice, it just means that it's the best you've seen thus far. Go ahead and read the next choice. If the next choice is worse than the one you've already selected, keep going to the next answer choice. If the next choice is better than the choice you've already selected, mentally mark the new answer choice as your best guess.

The first answer choice that you select becomes your standard. Every other answer choice must be benchmarked against that standard. That choice is correct until proven otherwise by another answer choice beating it out. Once you've decided that no other answer choice seems as good, do one final check to ensure that your answer choice answers the question posed.

Valid Information

Don't discount any of the information provided in the question. Every piece of information may be necessary to determine the correct answer. None of the information in the question is there to throw you off (while the answer choices will certainly have information to throw you off). If two seemingly unrelated topics are discussed, don't ignore either. You can be confident there is a relationship, or it wouldn't be included in the question, and you are probably going to have to determine what that relationship is to find the answer.

Avoid "Fact Traps"

Don't get distracted by a choice that is factually true. Your search is for the answer that answers the question. Stay focused and don't fall for an answer that is true but incorrect. Always go back to the question and make sure you're choosing an answer that actually answers the question and is not just a true statement. An answer can be factually correct, but it MUST answer the question asked. Additionally, two answers can both be seemingly correct, so be sure to read all of the answer choices, and make sure that you get the one that BEST answers the question.

Milk the Question

Some of the questions may throw you completely off. They might deal with a subject you have not been exposed to, or one that you haven't reviewed in years. While your lack of knowledge about the subject will be a hindrance, the question itself can give you many clues that will help you find the correct answer. Read the question carefully and look for clues. Watch particularly for adjectives and nouns describing difficult terms or words that you don't recognize. Regardless of if you completely understand a word or not, replacing it with a synonym either provided or one you more familiar with may help you to understand what the questions are asking. Rather than wracking your mind about specific detailed information concerning a difficult term or word, try to use mental substitutes that are easier to understand.

The Trap of Familiarity

Don't just choose a word because you recognize it. On difficult questions, you may not recognize a number of words in the answer choices. The test writers don't put "make-believe" words on the test; so don't think that just because you only recognize all the words in one answer choice means that answer choice must be correct. If you only recognize words in one answer choice, then focus on that one. Is it correct? Try your best to determine if it is correct. If it is, that is great, but if it doesn't, eliminate it. Each word and answer choice you eliminate increases your chances of getting the question correct, even if you then have to guess among the unfamiliar choices.

Eliminate Answers

Eliminate choices as soon as you realize they are wrong. But be careful! Make sure you consider all of the possible answer choices. Just because one appears right, doesn't mean that the next one won't be even better! The test writers will usually put more than one good answer choice for every question, so read all of them. Don't worry if you are stuck between two that seem right. By getting down to just two remaining possible choices, your odds are now 50/50. Rather than wasting too much time, play the odds. You are guessing, but guessing wisely, because you've been able to knock out some of the answer choices that you know are wrong. If you are eliminating choices and realize that the last answer choice you are left with is also obviously wrong, don't panic. Start over and consider each choice again. There may easily be something that you missed the first time and will realize on the second pass.

Tough Questions

If you are stumped on a problem or it appears too hard or too difficult, don't waste time. Move on! Remember though, if you can quickly check for obviously incorrect answer choices, your chances of guessing correctly are greatly improved. Before you completely give up, at least try to knock out a couple of possible answers. Eliminate what you can and then guess at the remaining answer choices before moving on.

Brainstorm

If you get stuck on a difficult question, spend a few seconds quickly brainstorming. Run through the complete list of possible answer choices. Look at each choice and ask yourself, "Could this answer the question satisfactorily?" Go through each answer choice and consider it independently of the other. By systematically going through all possibilities, you may find something that you would otherwise overlook. Remember that when you get stuck, it's important to try to keep moving.

Read Carefully

Understand the problem. Read the question and answer choices carefully. Don't miss the question because you misread the terms. You have plenty of time to read each question thoroughly and make sure you understand what is being asked. Yet a happy medium must be attained, so don't waste too much time. You must read carefully, but efficiently.

Face Value

When in doubt, use common sense. Always accept the situation in the problem at face value. Don't read too much into it. These problems will not require you to make huge leaps of logic. The test writers aren't trying to throw you off with a cheap trick. If you have to go beyond creativity and make a leap of logic in order to have an answer choice answer the question, then you should look at the other answer choices. Don't overcomplicate the problem by creating theoretical relationships or explanations that will warp time or space. These are normal problems rooted in reality. It's just that the applicable relationship or explanation may not be readily apparent and you have to figure things out. Use your common sense to interpret anything that isn't clear.

Prefixes

If you're having trouble with a word in the question or answer choices, try dissecting it. Take advantage of every clue that the word might include. Prefixes and suffixes can be a huge help. Usually they allow you to determine a basic meaning. Pre- means before, post- means after, pro - is positive, de- is negative. From these prefixes and suffixes, you can get an idea of the general meaning of the word and try to put it into context. Beware though of any traps. Just because con is the opposite of pro, doesn't necessarily mean congress is the opposite of progress!

Hedge Phrases

Watch out for critical "hedge" phrases, such as likely, may, can, will often, sometimes, often, almost, mostly, usually, generally, rarely, sometimes. Question writers insert these hedge phrases to cover every possibility. Often an answer choice will be wrong simply because it leaves no room for exception. Avoid answer choices that have definitive words like "exactly," and "always".

Switchback Words

Stay alert for "switchbacks". These are the words and phrases frequently used to alert you to shifts in thought. The most common switchback word is "but". Others include although, however, nevertheless, on the other hand, even though, while, in spite of, despite, regardless of.

New Information

Correct answer choices will rarely have completely new information included. Answer choices typically are straightforward reflections of the material asked about and will directly relate to the question. If a new piece of information is included in an answer choice that doesn't even seem to relate to the topic being asked about, then that answer choice is likely incorrect. All of the information needed to answer the question is usually provided for you, and so you should not have to make guesses that are unsupported or choose answer choices that require unknown information that cannot be reasoned on its own.

Time Management

On technical questions, don't get lost on the technical terms. Don't spend too much time on any one question. If you don't know what a term means, then since you don't have a dictionary, odds are you aren't going to get much further. You should immediately recognize terms as whether or not you know them. If you don't, work with the other clues that you have, the other answer choices and terms provided, but don't waste too much time trying to figure out a difficult term.

Contextual Clues

Look for contextual clues. An answer can be right but not correct. The contextual clues will help you find the answer that is most right and is correct. Understand the context in which a phrase or statement is made. This will help you make important distinctions.

Don't Panic

Panicking will not answer any questions for you. Therefore, it isn't helpful. When you first see the question, if your mind goes blank, take a deep breath. Force yourself to mechanically go through the steps of solving the problem and using the strategies you've learned.

Pace Yourself

Don't get clock fever. It's easy to be overwhelmed when you're looking at a page full of questions, your mind is full of random thoughts and feeling confused, and the clock is ticking down faster than you would like. Calm down and maintain the pace that you have set for yourself. As long as you are on track by monitoring your pace, you are guaranteed to have enough time for yourself. When you get to the last few minutes of the test, it may seem like you won't have enough time left, but if you only have as many questions as you should have left at that point, then you're right on track!

Answer Selection

The best way to pick an answer choice is to eliminate all of those that are wrong, until only one is left and confirm that is the correct answer. Sometimes though, an answer choice may immediately look right. Be careful! Take a second to make sure that the other choices are not equally obvious. Don't make a hasty mistake. There are only two times that you should stop before checking other answers. First is when you are positive that the answer choice you have selected is correct. Second is when time is almost out and you have to make a quick guess!

Check Your Work

Since you will probably not know every term listed and the answer to every question, it is important that you get credit for the ones that you do know. Don't miss any questions through careless mistakes. If at all possible, try to take a second to look back over your answer selection and make sure you've selected the correct answer choice and haven't made a costly careless mistake (such as marking an answer choice that you didn't mean to mark). This quick double check should more than pay for itself in caught mistakes for the time it costs.

Beware of Directly Quoted Answers

Sometimes an answer choice will repeat word for word a portion of the question or reference section. However, beware of such exact duplication – it may be a trap! More than likely, the correct choice will paraphrase or summarize a point, rather than being exactly the same wording.

Slang

Scientific sounding answers are better than slang ones. An answer choice that begins "To compare the outcomes..." is much more likely to be correct than one that begins "Because some people insisted..."

Extreme Statements

Avoid wild answers that throw out highly controversial ideas that are proclaimed as established fact. An answer choice that states the "process should be used in certain situations, if..." is much more likely to be correct than one that states the "process should be discontinued completely." The first is a calm rational statement and doesn't even make a definitive, uncompromising stance, using a hedge word "if" to provide wiggle room, whereas the second choice is a radical idea and far more extreme.

Answer Choice Families

When you have two or more answer choices that are direct opposites or parallels, one of them is usually the correct answer. For instance, if one answer choice states "x increases" and another answer choice states "x decreases" or "y increases," then those two or three answer choices are very similar in construction and fall into the same family of answer choices. A family of answer choices is when two or three answer choices are very similar in construction, and yet often have a directly opposite meaning. Usually the correct answer choice will be in that family of answer choices. The "odd man out" or answer choice that doesn't seem to fit the parallel construction of the other answer choices is more likely to be incorrect.

Special Report: Additional Bonus Material

Due to our efforts to try to keep this book to a manageable length, we've created a link that will give you access to all of your additional bonus material.

Please visit http://www.mometrix.com/bonus948/cnrn to access the information.